Contents

About the Title...

The title of this book, *The Lost Chord*, is derived from a legend about the composer and organist Alexander Scriabin. According to the legend, Scriabin was composing at the organ when he played a chord that was so powerful that, for an instant, he was transfixed by its sound—it was the musical manifestation of The Truth. For the rest of his life he sought to find the chord again, but never did.

This legend beautifully illustrates the power of music. Most of us have had an experience with music that has touched us in some way. Perhaps you know a song that, when you hear it, reminds you of someone who is special to you or of an experience that is important to you. Remember Humphrey Bogart and Ingrid Bergman in *Casablanca* and their response to "As Time Goes By"?

William Sears, a music therapy researcher, coined the phrase "extramusical associations" to explain this phenomenon: music's ability to transport the listener or performer to another time and place. This close association of music with memory is one of the reasons that music can be so powerful for persons with Alzheimer's disease or related dementias.

In an article for the magazine *Aging*, Laura Paulman cites Dr. Robert Katzman of the Albert Einstein School of Medicine as saying that "...the portions of the brain that respond to music are the last to deteriorate in illnesses affecting the brain. Consequently, music and singing are suggested treatments to help people with Alzheimer's."

Since this article was published, there has been much interest in developing music programs for persons with dementia. *The Lost Chord* was written to assist the family or professional caregiver in providing quality musical experiences. The first part of this book focuses on the special needs of this population; the second part contains suggested music activities appropriate for individuals in the different stages of dementia. My hope is that this book will help to bring music into the lives of people with dementia by "de-mystifying" it, and will provide music group descriptions that anyone can follow. You don't need to be a musician to provide quality music groups.

I do wish to issue one caveat. What I am providing in this book are music group descriptions. I feel that quality music groups can be provided by anyone who is interested enough in music to want to use it in his/her work. What this book will *not* do is to train you to be a music therapist. In the United States, music therapists have graduated from degree programs in music therapy that are approved by either the National Association for Music Therapy or the American Association for Music Therapy, and have met the requirements for registration or certification from these organizations. For more information on the training of music therapists and the field of music therapy, you can write to the National Association for Music Therapy, Inc., or the American Association for Music Therapy, Inc. (See Appendix, page 95, for addresses.)

It is my sincere hope that this book will encourage you to add music to your day and that the experience will be positive and just plain fun for everyone involved.

Musically Yours,

Melanie Chavin
June 1991

Introduction

"Isn't it depressing, working with Alzheimer's patients?"... "How can you stand doing what you do?"

♪

Caregivers of persons with Alzheimer's disease and related dementias are often faced with questions like these. Usually, these questions are followed by a statement such as, "I could *never* do that!" or "You must be a saint." It's difficult for those with no experience in living with or assisting persons with dementia to understand the problems and the rewards that accompany this vocation.

In the future, more and more of us will become caregivers of those with dementing illnesses. According to a 1989 study done by Denis Evans, M.D., the incidence of Alzheimer's disease and related dementias may be as high as 47 percent in persons over the age of eighty-five. This means that many of us may eventually develop dementia. Is this cause for alarm? Certainly. But more than that, it is a call for those of us that will be fortunate enough to escape this disease to become adept at living with and caring for those persons who are not so fortunate.

The health care community has come a long way in understanding the special needs of persons with dementia, but it still has a long way to go. On the one hand, hospitals, adult day care centers, and long-term care facilities are showing more interest in the concept of special care units for persons with dementia. On the other hand, many facilities interpret this to mean simply segregating persons with dementia from the rest of the facility's population, with no special training for staff and no special programming for the residents. The result? Anxious, agitated residents and a battle-weary staff.

What I hope this book will do is help you to understand dementia from the point of view of the person with dementia. A book full of music groups won't help you if you don't have a basic understanding of how dementing illnesses affect people.

For the past several years, I've worked as a music therapist and program coordinator at the Alzheimer's Family Care Center (AFCC), a dementia-specific adult day care center located in Chicago, Illinois. This program serves people of varying cognitive levels, from persons who have recently been diagnosed to those who are well into the later stages of a dementing illness.

I've learned so much from our clients. The importance of nonverbal communication was taught to me by those persons who can no longer communicate in traditional ways. From those who need more time to process communication and information than I do, I've learned to slow down. I've learned to react calmly to difficult situations, since anxious, frightened, or angry people tend to take their emotional cues from the people around them. Most of all, I have learned to be flexible and to take the client's lead.

What does this mean, "taking the client's lead"? When I first worked with persons with dementia, I became frustrated because I was accustomed to "being in charge." My training was based on behavioral theory, that states that all behavior is learned and that the therapist's task is to help the patient to change faulty behaviors into more appropriate behaviors. This theory makes sense if you are working with persons who have the capacity to learn. Persons with dementia may lack this capacity. They cannot change their behavior for the long term. It is those of us who live and work with these persons who need to do the changing.

Once I understood this, working with persons with dementia became much easier. I learned that sometimes my group plans clashed with the needs of the participants. If I plan a discussion/reminiscence group when the clients want to sing, then forging ahead with my original plan will just frustrate the group (and me). If my goal is to have an individual strum the autoharp but she wants to listen to me play, then there's no sense in my risking a catastrophic reaction from her by insisting that she do what I want her to do. Consequently, I still try new things, and sometimes they work well. But I've learned to ask myself, "Whose needs are being met by this activity? The clients' or my own?"

Music can at times be overstimulating for persons with dementia and is not appropriate for all persons at all times. If an individual has never liked music, the chances are that s/he will not enjoy it now either. If a person never liked a particular style of music, s/he will probably not like it now. Playing "calming" music for an anxious or agitated person may actually increase the anxiety if the anxiety is due to overstimulation. Remember that sometimes "silence is golden."

The most important lesson that I have learned is this: the person with dementia is still a person. Even after the disease has taken its toll by robbing the person of most of his/her intellectual and physical capacities, there's a person in there. One of the most rewarding experiences a caregiver can have is seeing a glimpse of the individual's personality shining through the dementia. This is truly a triumph of the human spirit.

Part I

The Person with Dementia

Chapter 1

A Brief Overview of Alzheimer's Disease and Other Dementing Illnesses

"Is Alzheimer's disease the same as senility?"... "You never used to hear about Alzheimer's disease. Is it something new?"... "How do you know if you've got Alzheimer's? I mean, don't we all get forgetful when we get old?"... "Why do you use the term 'dementia' when you talk about these patients? Doesn't 'dementia' mean the same thing as 'crazy'?"

♪

These are the questions I'm asked the most frequently when I give presentations or tell people what I do. They're good questions and reflect the confusion that many of us have about these diseases and the terminology surrounding them.

Let's start with the first question. According to the fourteenth edition of *Taber's Cyclopedic Medical Dictionary*, senility is defined as "mental or physical weakness that may be associated with old age." As we age, we normally have increased difficulty with memory and recall. But these memory problems are transient in nature and not so severe as to cause major difficulties. The technical term for these memory lapses is "benign transient senescence," and we've all experienced it: forgetting where we put the car keys, suddenly forgetting the name of someone we've known for a long time, losing our train of thought in the middle of a sentence. This is perfectly normal.

In contrast, Alzheimer's disease and related dementias are much more serious than this. The memory loss is progressive and irreversible. Major changes in behavior may occur and the individual's judgment is impaired. This is a disease process and is in no way a normal part of aging.

Although we hear more about Alzheimer's disease (AD) now than we did in the past, it is not a new disease. AD was first described in 1907 by Alois Alzheimer, a German physician. He noticed the symptoms of progressive memory loss in a fifty-year-old woman. Since the conventional wisdom at that time was that memory loss was a normal part of aging (senility), he called the condition "pre-senile dementia." We now know that the condition Dr. Alzheimer saw in his fifty-year-old patient is the same condition that occurs in persons age sixty-five and older.

AD is no more common now than in Dr. Alzheimer's day. It's simply that, with all of the medical advances that we have seen in this century, people are living longer. Many people do not begin to show signs of dementia until they are in their seventies or eighties. Years ago, many of these persons may have died of other causes before the dementia showed up.

When physicians and health care professionals use the word "dementia" to describe AD and related disorders, they are referring to a group of symptoms that is earmarked by the reduction of intellectual capacities and the deterioration of mental state associated with organic brain disease. The person isn't "crazy"—s/he has a disease that causes memory loss.

Not all dementias are permanent and irreversible. There are some medical conditions that cause dementia that disappear once the condition is treated. Some of these reversible causes of dementia are drug toxicity, dehydration, thyroid disease, vitamin deficiencies, renal disease, and severe depression. When an older person begins to show symptoms of dementia, it's always important to have a full medical evaluation done so that reversible causes can be detected and treated.

If an irreversible dementia is suspected, the physician may want to do further testing, as there are several diseases that cause irreversible dementia. Each of these conditions has its own set of symptoms and suggested treatments, so it's important to determine the exact disease.

Alzheimer's disease (AD) is diagnosed by ruling out all other causes of dementia. At this time, AD cannot be definitively diagnosed until the person dies and a brain autopsy is performed. Even then the diagnosis isn't sure, as autopsies are only 85 percent accurate. Unfortunately, many persons who are diagnosed with AD haven't received a full medical workup, so their dementia may be due to another cause. It is very important to insist on full neurological testing before accepting the diagnosis of AD since some of the other dementias require medical treatment to prevent unnecessary deterioration.

The symptoms of AD vary from case to case depending upon a number of factors including age of onset, the individual's general physical condition, the individual's personality before the onset of the illness, and his/her medical and psychological history. Researchers have described anywhere from three to seven stages of the disease in an effort to describe its course in a concise way. In reality, few persons progress neatly through these stages, which makes it extremely difficult to pinpoint exactly which stage a person is in.

Current research is beginning to focus on the concept that AD may actually be a group of diseases rather than one disease. Some cases of AD seem to be genetic, with a clear familial history of the disease. Some people develop the disease before the age of sixty-five while others don't exhibit symptoms until they are in their seventies or eighties. Researchers are also looking at the chemical changes in the brains of AD patients and are testing drugs to see if these changes can be controlled or reversed. Diagnostic tools are being tested, with the hope that early detection of the disease may be helpful in treating it.

Multi-infarct dementia (MID) is caused by "mini-strokes" that may or may not impair the individual physically but that cause cognitive dysfunction. Persons with MID often have medical problems associated with an increased risk for strokes including diabetes, hypertension, and atherosclerosis. Persons with MID may show fluctuations in their dementia and may occasionally have physical symptoms of strokes (weakness on one side, difficulty with swallowing, slurred speech, incontinence). Often, these strokes are very mild and the person recovers quickly from them; however, each new stroke leaves the person with some residual physical and cognitive damage. Each case of MID is different: some people have strokes very infrequently and manage to stay at the same physical and cognitive level for some time; others have strokes often and become quite debilitated.

A small percentage of **Parkinson's Disease** patients eventually develop dementia. Some Parkinson's patients are mistakenly labeled as having dementia because of their slow response time when answering questions and because of the blank, staring facial expression that is a hallmark of the disease. If the person with Parkinson's does have dementia, it's important for the caregiver to sort out which behaviors are due to the dementia and which are due to the physical demands of the disease. For example, if the person doesn't respond right away to questions or commands, it may be due to the individual's rigidity or other physical demands of the disease, rather than to the dementia.

There are many other diseases that cause dementia. The bibliography in the back of this book lists several books that discuss these diseases in more detail. If you want more information on Alzheimer's disease and related illnesses, or on support services that may be available to you, please contact:

The Alzheimer's Association
919 N. Michigan Avenue, Suite 1000
Chicago, Illinois 60611-1676
312-853-3060

Currently, AD and related dementias are the fourth leading cause of death among older adults in the United States. Although there is no cure for these diseases, there are ways that we can help to improve the quality of life for these persons. The chapters that follow discuss ways that we, the caregivers, can help persons with dementia to achieve their full potential.

Chapter 2

Common Behaviors and How to Work with Them

Anxiety

Mrs. M was sitting in the music group, wringing her hands and looking quite anxious. "What should I do?" she asked the music therapist. This question was followed by several more: "How will I get home?" "Where is my husband?" "Do you know me? Am I OK?" The music therapist answered her questions and Mrs. M appeared to be reassured. The music therapist resumed the music activity. A few minutes later, Mrs. M began again: "What should I do?"

Mrs. F was participating in the exercise group. About 15 minutes into the group, she stood up and walked out of the room. When she came back a few minutes later, she was wearing her coat. The group leader encouraged her to take her coat off, as it was very warm in the room, but Mrs. F refused. After this, Mrs. F left the room every five minutes or so, walked to the front door, looked out of the window, and then returned to the group. The group leader was unable to convince Mrs. F to stay in her seat.

Mrs. V and her caregiver were preparing lunch when Mrs. V suddenly put down the bread she had been buttering and walked to the kitchen door. She could not open it and asked her caregiver, "Please open the door." The caregiver tried to distract Mrs. V from the door and encouraged her to continue assisting with lunch, but Mrs. V became even more persistent. After several minutes of this, Mrs. V became angry and said, "I need to go now!" and pushed the caregiver out of her way.

♪

These examples of anxious behavior should sound familiar to caregivers of persons with dementia. Anxiety often seems to come out of nowhere, and it's difficult to find a way to refocus the person back to what they were doing before they became anxious. What do you do when the person with whom you're working becomes anxious?

Try to think about a time when you've been anxious. How did you feel in that situation? Were you nervous? Did you have a hard time concentrating? Was it difficult for you to breathe? Were you shaky?

Each of us reacts differently to anxiety. When I'm anxious, it helps me to be alone for a while, to pace a bit and to collect my thoughts. I become annoyed with talkative people. A friend of mine is exactly the opposite. When she's anxious, she likes to be with other people; she says it calms her down to talk to someone. You may have a different way of coping with anxiety. The point is, each one of us is an individual and has our own way of dealing with anxiety-provoking situations.

People with dementia each have their own way of dealing with anxiety as well. While some people may respond well to distraction, others may become more anxious when their questions aren't answered (like Mrs. M). Mrs. F paces when anxious, but does not become angry or agitated. The pacing itself seems to calm her. Mrs. V paces when anxious, but becomes agitated and clearly needs more than verbal reassurance. Here we have three women, all with dementia, all anxious, but all requiring different interventions to reduce their anxiety level.

The above examples are real ones. These incidents occurred at the AFCC, and as you've probably guessed, I was the caregiver in them. I didn't deal with these situations especially well at the time, but as I came to know these women I learned a bit about their coping styles.

Mrs. M's anxiety came from not knowing where she was or how she was going to get home. She was looking for reassurance and a sense of security. This is a very common theme among persons with dementia who may be "looking for home" even when they are at home. The person may ask for her/his mother, spouse, sibling, or a close friend.

Try to imagine being in the shoes of a person with dementia. Mrs. M is anxious because she doesn't know where she is or who she's with. She's in a room with six other people. Five of them are older adults. The sixth is a younger woman who is sitting next to her in the circle, playing a guitar and encouraging the group to sing and play rhythm instruments. Can you imagine what's going through Mrs. M's mind?:

"Where the heck am I? This isn't home. We don't do this at home. Do I know any of these people? No, I don't. Where's my husband? Do I live here now? What is this thing I'm holding and what am I supposed to do with it? That girl looks like she's in charge. I'll ask her what I'm doing here. I wish she'd stop singing and talk to me!"

♪

Music is an enjoyable experience for most of us, but in this case Mrs. M's mind was clearly on more important things. By continuing to encourage Mrs. M to participate in the music group, I was adding to her confusion and stress.

If I were running this music group today, I'd ask my co-leader to take Mrs. M outside of the group for a few minutes because she needed reassurance, not music. If I didn't have a co-leader, I'd end the music group because Mrs. M's anxiety could lead to a catastrophic reaction if I continued to ignore it. It's also possible that the music was too stimulating for her at that moment.

Like Mrs. M, Mrs. F was anxious to go home, but she wasn't verbal and couldn't tell me what she wanted. If I had paid more attention to her nonverbal communication, I may have figured out what she was saying: "I'm not sure of the routine here or if I can trust you. I think it's time to go home. I'll walk to the front door every few minutes to check to see if my husband is here yet."

Mrs. F continues to put on her coat before the exercise group and we've learned to accept this; wearing the coat helps her to feel more secure. She has become accustomed to the routine and she knows that her husband picks her up later in the afternoon. She doesn't start pacing to and from the door until after lunch. Mrs. F's pacing doesn't disrupt the group and she participates in it between her trips to the door. We've learned to adjust to her routine. We know that if we try to prevent her from pacing or if we try to wrestle her coat away from her, she'll become too anxious to participate in the group.

Mrs. V enjoys helping with what we call "normalization activities": tasks that are meaningful, appropriate, and that contribute to the day-to-day routine at the day center. In particular, she assists with folding the napkins for lunch, serving snacks, wiping off the tables, and sorting the utensils. She is also able to assist with meal preparation, including buttering the bread we serve with lunch. In performing these tasks, she is quite high-functioning.

Mrs. V is prone to episodes of anxiety, however. When she becomes anxious, efforts to engage her in activities, even those which she is able to perform under normal circumstances, are futile. Distraction does not work for her, nor do efforts to calm her through verbal reassurance. The only effective way to reduce Mrs. V's anxiety is to take her for a walk outside of the building.

We learned this by accident. Mrs. V is Greek and speaks a mixture of Greek and English. Although she continues to comprehend English, she primarily communicates in Greek. After one especially difficult afternoon for her, a staff member asked her daughter to translate a phrase she'd said over and over that day. It turned out to be, "I want to get some fresh air." It seems that Mrs. V had been a rancher when she was younger and she was unaccustomed to being cooped up indoors all day. The staff began to take her for walks when she became especially anxious and these walks helped to calm her.

Becoming sensitive to anxiety-producing situations is one of the first steps in heading off catastrophic reactions. It's important to recognize that when a person with dementia does something unusual or is unable to perform a task, s/he is not being difficult. It's a symptom of the disease, and you can be sure that it's just as upsetting for him/her as it is for you.

Catastrophic Reactions

It's important to deal with anxiety as soon as possible because, unchecked, it can lead to catastrophic reactions. Catastrophic reactions are overreactions to situations and can result in anger, crying, or agitation in the person. These reactions don't necessarily lead to violent behavior, but this can occur.

Once the catastrophic reaction has begun, it is difficult to stop it; you may need to simply ride it out, while making sure that the individual is safe. Let's look at a few examples of catastrophic reactions and how to deal with them.

Mrs. Z lived with her daughter, Gina, and her son-in-law, Fred. In the evening, Mrs. Z would occasionally begin to ask for her mother and would want to go to her mother's house (her mother had been deceased for some time). Gina could usually redirect Mrs. Z and head off a catastrophic reaction. One night Mrs. Z became very angry and paranoid, accusing Gina and Fred of "keeping me from my mother." Mrs. Z got dressed, put on her coat, and pushed past Gina and Fred to get outside. Gina went after her mother, but Mrs. Z walked quickly and shouted at Gina to get away every time she caught up with her.

♪

What would you do if you were Gina?

Mrs. Z was very angry. She didn't respond to Gina's efforts to redirect her. Gina did the only thing she could: she followed Mrs. Z at a safe distance until she became tired and cold and was ready to go home. Mrs. Z effectively "walked off" her anger.

But not all catastrophic reactions end this easily:

Mr. T, an AD patient, was a participant in an adult day center. When he became anxious, he would insist on taking walks outside of the building. Unfortunately, the walks did not help to calm him. He'd become very angry at the staff person who was with him and would try to run away. On one occasion, the police had to be called because the day center staff feared for Mr. T's safety. He was so upset that it was feared he might run into traffic, board a bus, or jump into a stranger's car.

♪

In situations like this the best thing to do is to stay with the person until help arrives, be it additional staff persons, family members, or, in extreme cases, the police. In most instances it's possible to head off catastrophic reactions before they get out of hand.

Catastrophic reactions occur when the person feels that s/he is no longer in control of a situation. Think of how you'd feel if no one would let you leave the house. I know I'd be angry and probably paranoid if someone was always watching me.

It's not always possible to head off catastrophic reactions. One way to try to prevent them is to be sensitive to the person's anxiety level and to work to eliminate the anxiety before a catastrophic reaction occurs. If a reaction occurs despite your best efforts to avert it, remember these pointers:

1. **Examine the environment.** If the reaction is clearly in response to something in the environment, try to remove the offending stimulus or take the individual to a calmer place.

2. **Remain calm.** If you appear anxious or angry, the person with dementia will react in this way too.

3. **Have a backup system in place.** If possible, let someone know that there is a problem and that you may need help. (In Mr. T's case, we'd tell a co-worker, "I'm going on a walk with Mr. T. If we're not back in 15 minutes, start looking for us." We've since purchased mobile telephones so that we can call for assistance, if needed.)

4. **Reassure the person.** Speak in a comforting (but not condescending) tone, and let the person know that you are there to help: "I know that you're upset—is there anything that I can do to help?"

5. **Reassure yourself.** The catastrophic reaction won't last forever. It will end eventually.

6. **The reaction is not necessarily your fault.** Sometimes, despite your best intentions, the person with dementia may misinterpret something and become upset.

Catastrophic reactions are frightening for both the caregiver and the person experiencing them. When I become frustrated with a person who's having a catastrophic reaction, I try to remember what I heard from an AFCC client after she'd had a minor catastrophic reaction at the day center: "I know what I did doesn't make sense, but I can't help it. I'm sorry. Thank you for putting up with me."

Overstimulation

You and I have the ability to screen sensory stimulation; we can pay attention to some things in the environment while we ignore others. The person with dementia may become confused by competing sensory stimulation and can become anxious as a result.

If the person with whom you are working seems anxious for no apparent reason, take a good look at the environment:

1. **Is it too crowded?** Some individuals become anxious in large groups of people or in cluttered areas. There may be too much to look at or too many things to negotiate around.

2. **Is it too noisy?** If you're trying to engage the person in an activity or task when there's a television playing, the television will win out every time (as will the radio, the public address system, the ringing telephone, the stereo, etc.).

3. **Is it too busy?** It's difficult for persons with dementia to concentrate on a task or a conversation if there is too much unrelated activity going on around them.

4. **Is the environment too visually stimulating?** In our zeal to provide sensory stimulation, we may actually overstimulate persons with dementia:

While sitting in his usual seat at the day center, Mr. J began to react oddly to a newly-decorated bulletin board. He looked concerned and began to fidget in his seat. The therapist asked what was troubling him. "Did I do something wrong?" he asked. The therapist replied, "Not at all. What makes you think you did something wrong?" "Well," he said, pointing at the bulletin board, "I'm in jail!"

♪

The bulletin board that Mr. J was facing was decorated with the caption, "At the Zoo," and had photos of various zoo animals on it. It was covered with one-inch strips of black construction paper placed about six inches apart to simulate the bars of a cage. Mr. J's misinterpretation of the bulletin board was certainly understandable.

The sense of hearing is the most overstimulated sense in the majority of homes and institutions. We've become accustomed to having the radio or television on even if no one is paying attention to it. American society is a noisy one!

But sound is very distracting to the person with dementia, who may have difficulty focusing on your voice if there is another sound source nearby: "Do I listen to the TV or to my daughter? Which of these sounds that I hear is my daughter?"

If you're trying to get the attention of a person with dementia, make sure you're not competing with someone or something else. Turn off the television and the radio. Try to go to a quiet place. If you're trying to encourage the person to participate in an activity or task in the middle of a confusing, noisy environment, you have little chance of success.

It's impossible to screen out all distracters, but a bit of creativity can help to keep them within manageable limits. The AFCC had a "doorbell problem": when it rang, our clients became preoccupied with it. One of the staff came upon the idea of muting the doorbell by stuffing paper in the mechanism. The result? The doorbell still rings, but quietly; the clients often don't notice it over the sounds of the group.

The following suggestions may be helpful in developing a calm environment:

1. **Make it quiet.** Unplug nearby telephones, turn down the ringer, or have someone take messages for you during the activity or task. You may also consider using an answering machine to pick up calls (set it to pick up after one ring). If you work in an institution that utilizes public address pages, try to work in an area that isn't affected by the pages, or see if the pages can be held for the duration of the activity.

2. **Look at the lighting.** Is the room too bright or too dim? You can't get the person's attention if s/he can't see you. If sunlight or glare is streaming in through a window, close the drapes or pull the shades. If the room is too dim, brighten it.

3. **Watch your voice tone.** If you consistently talk too loudly or have an anxious or annoyed tone to your voice, the person with dementia will respond accordingly.

4. **Avoid distractions.** If possible, work in a room where the door can be closed so that the person/group isn't distracted by interruptions or activity outside of the room. Make sure that others know not to disturb you.

5. **Be gentle and patient.** More than once a well-meaning caregiver has overstimulated a person with dementia by startling him/her, giving too many instructions, or not giving enough time to respond.

Try to remember a time when you've felt overstimulated. I remember feeling overstimulated by a high school algebra tutor who was miles ahead of me in mathematical knowledge. He interpreted my silences as intelligent broodings on the laws of mathematics when they were really desperate attempts to grasp the basic concepts of algebra. He'd be off and running on the next concept when I was struggling to understand the last one, and my brain would reel from trying to sort out all of the things he was telling me. I try to remember this feeling when I'm working with a person who is having difficulty understanding something; a bit of patience and empathy goes a long way.

Reduced Attention Span

One of the biggest challenges that caregivers of persons with dementia face is the reduced attention span that is characteristic of dementing illnesses. People with dementia are often easily distracted, which makes it difficult for them to concentrate on an activity or task for more than a few minutes.

Controlling for potential distracters in the environment, as described above, can be extremely helpful. Additionally, it is important to plan several different ways of accomplishing activities and tasks:

Mr. C had a difficult time using utensils to feed himself. He ate with his hands and, as a result, often made quite a mess and missed eating a good portion of his food. The day center staff first tried giving him verbal cues to pick up his fork, place it in his food, etc. When verbal cues didn't help, physical cues were tried: putting the fork into Mr. C's hand and guiding the fork into the food, then into his mouth. Finally, adaptive equipment was used. Mr. C was unable to master any of these techniques, despite one-to-one training by day center staff.

♪

In the above example, Mr. C became so distracted with doing what the staff wanted him to do (eat with utensils) that he could no longer figure out how to get food into his mouth. *His* major goal was to eat; at this time, ours was to get him to eat *properly*. We had little success until the day his wife informed us that he'd been eating with his hands for some time now at home and was doing quite well, thank you! The staff abandoned the effort to get him to eat with utensils and began to make him sandwiches and finger foods for lunch. His nutritional intake improved considerably.

Mr. C had a reduced attention span, which interfered with his ability to learn new skills (such as using adaptive equipment). He was able to eat sandwiches because this didn't involve any new skills and, in fact, worked with an existing behavior (eating with his hands.)

People with dementia have dramatically shortened attention spans, so it is important to plan activities and tasks with this in mind. At the AFCC, we may set aside an hour and a half for an activity, but within that time we may have three or four short activities planned. For example, the AFCC schedules a current events group each morning for our higher-functioning clients. Do we discuss current events for the entire time? Of course not. The group plan may look like this:

1. **Greeting the group** (15 min.): small talk, discussion of the weather, reading the lunch menu, announcements, serving coffee.

2. **Current events** (15-20 min.): reading the newspaper headlines and discussing them, looking at the sports scores, reading the horoscopes for all of the group members, reading "Ann Landers" and "Dear Abby" and guessing at their advice.

3. **Word game** (10 min.): alphabet lists on a current event topic, seasonal theme, or upcoming holiday (for example, for the theme "America/Fourth of July": A = America, B = Baseball, C = Constitution, D = Declaration of Independence, etc.).

4. **Morning snack** (10 min.): a nutritious snack, accompanied by light discussion or "bounce questions" such as those in Mindstretchers (see bibliography.)

5. **Music** (10-15 min.): sing-along of songs chosen for their appropriateness to the season, upcoming holidays, or current events. For the "America/Fourth of July" theme we may sing songs such as "The Battle Hymn of the Republic," "My Country 'Tis of Thee," "America, the Beautiful," "The Star Spangled Banner," etc.

On paper, our current events group lasts an hour and a half. In reality, it is several shorter groups joined under the theme of "current events/orientation." This structure manages to meet the criteria for current events/reality orientation programming in a way that is sensitive to our clients' reduced attention spans.

Working with persons with a reduced attention span is difficult. Here are some points to remember:

1. **Simplify.** It's helpful to break down activities/tasks into several small steps. The person with dementia may not be able to complete an entire activity (such as making a sandwich) but may be able to remove two slices of bread from the package, place a slice of bread on a plate, and spread peanut butter on the slice of bread.

2. **Set realistic goals.** Rather than looking at success as the individual's active participation in an *entire* session, consider a session successful if a percentage of its steps are completed. (In the example of Mr. C, perhaps he didn't eat with adaptive equipment, but he did eat. This is success.)

3. **Be flexible.** Realize that the person(s) you're planning the session for may not want to do what you have planned. Consider how you'd feel if you wanted to vacation in Florida but ended up in Alaska: both places are interesting and enjoyable, but vastly different.

4. **Expect the unexpected.** Go into a session with several backup plans. This way, you won't be caught off guard if your original idea doesn't work.

5. **Be fearless.** Don't be afraid to try new things. Some things will go well; some won't. You'll never know if you don't try.

Wandering and Pacing

Mr. S was in constant motion at the day center. He would only sit for a few minutes at a time, even during meals. He spent most of his day slowly walking around the day center, stopping only to interact socially with other participants and staff. During music groups, Mr. S would walk up to the therapist and stand directly in front of her, swaying and vocalizing along with the music. Although his pacing behavior was not a problem for Mr. S, it did become a problem for the higher-functioning participants, who had difficulty understanding Mr. S's need to walk. Mr. S began to become upset at their comments towards him: "Why don't you sit down?" "What's the matter with that guy?

♪

Wandering and pacing are among the most difficult behaviors to work with for caregivers of persons with dementia. As the above example illustrates, these behaviors can also be difficult for the person who is experiencing them. It's difficult not to feel awkward, upset, and embarrassed when people around you are constantly commenting on your inability to sit still. It's even more difficult when the people around you insist that you try to sit down when it's apparent that you can't—or you wouldn't be pacing in the first place!

Wandering and pacing are not the same behavior. Wandering tends to be connected with looking for something: "I'm looking for my husband." "Have you seen my coat?" Wanderers also tend to have a difficult time being confined to a building or a room.

Mrs. Z, who was looking for her mother in an earlier example in this book, experienced wandering as a behavior. Persons who wander may leave the house to go on walks and then become lost; frequently, wandering is the symptom that makes families realize that their relative's confusion is more than just benign forgetfulness.

Pacing appears less purposeful on the surface. If you ask the pacing person if s/he needs something, s/he may not be able to articulate a need. The pacing itself fulfills some inner need.

Mr. K was a quiet, reserved man who had recently begun to attend the day center. He was pleasant and polite, but would periodically stand up in a group and excuse himself. One of the staff followed him out of the room one day and asked him, "Is there something you are looking for?" "No," he said. Thinking he may be too shy to ask, she asked, "Are you looking for the bathroom?" "No," he said, "I just... need to stretch."

♪

Mr. S and Mr. K both paced. Only Mr. S wandered, however. Mr. S would always make a beeline for an open door; Mr. K had no difficulty staying indoors and never attempted to leave the building.

It's also important to be able to distinguish the difference between normal pacing and agitated pacing. In normal pacing, the person does not appear to be distressed in any way. The person tends to walk at a normal, or even a slow, pace. S/he appears calm and may interact purposefully with others in the area. Agitated pacing is of a faster pace; at times, the person may even run. The person may appear anxious, angry, or fearful. Some kind of intervention is needed to prevent the onset of a catastrophic reaction:

Mrs. N became upset one afternoon at the day center, asking constantly, "How will I get home?" She began to walk quickly from door to door, checking to see if she recognized anyone near the doors. If she heard a telephone ringing, she'd yell, "Is it for me?" It became apparent that she needed some reassurance, so a staff member wrote her a note that said, "Nancy will pick you up here at 4:00. Please wait for her." The staff member spent a few minutes with her, reassuring her that she would be picked up by Nancy (her daughter-in-law) at 4:00. Mrs. N continued to pace and express her concerns that she would not be able to get home. The staff member then called Nancy at work, explained the situation, and asked Nancy if she would talk to Mrs. N for a moment to reassure her. After the telephone call, Mrs. N was satisfied that she would get home safely and sat near the door waiting for Nancy to arrive.

♪

Mrs. N was experiencing agitated pacing on this day. It took a staff person 15 minutes to settle her down. It could be argued that 15 minutes spent away from the rest of the day center participants is too much time to spend on one person. However, if this 15 minutes was not spent on Mrs. N, a catastrophic reaction may have occurred that involved two or three staff persons and a considerably longer amount of time to resolve. Also, since Mrs. N was anxious but not agitated for the rest of the day, this was 15 minutes well-spent. It's much easier to spend a short period of time helping a person than a long period of time calming a person.

Most caregivers know that trying to get a wandering or pacing person to sit down simply isn't effective. This intervention brings to mind the saying, "Never try to teach a pig to sing. It wastes your time and annoys the pig."

At the AFCC, the persons for whom wandering or pacing are a *primary* behavior are included in a program that is called "The Walking Club." This program is held in a large room (approximately 20' x 20') and usually does not include more than eight participants at a time, with two staff members (one to run activities and interact with the participants; one to help with personal care and assist the group leader). Since everyone in the group has a need to move about, there is little conflict between the group members. For the persons for whom wandering/pacing is not a primary behavior, but instead an indication of intense anxiety, fear, or anger, the underlying issues that are causing the behavior are dealt with. In Mrs. K's case, she was reassured by knowing that she would get home safely. In Mrs. V's case, "getting fresh air" was a help to her. In Mrs. Z's case, the walk helped to distract her from her initial anger.

Although it is difficult to work or live with a person who is constantly in motion, it is important for caregivers to learn to accept the wandering or pacing person's need to move about. Forcing the person to sit down may cause a catastrophic reaction. Instead, use your imagination to find ways to adapt to the person's need to move around:

Mrs. L was in motion nearly all day. She would sit for only a few minutes at a time and spent the majority of the day walking slowly around the Walking Club area. This did not present a problem until mealtimes, since Mrs. L could not sit long enough to finish a meal. She would take a bite or two of her lunch and then walk away from the table, becoming angry when the staff would attempt to redirect her to her plate. The staff person who usually served Mrs. L lunch suggested giving her sandwiches, as she could eat them as she walked about. When this was done, Mrs. L's nutritional intake improved.

♪

Creativity is certainly the key to working with a person who is in constant motion. The AFCC has one Walking Club member (Mrs. G) who is not only constantly moving but also has a very short attention span. The most difficult part of the day for her is putting on her coat to leave at the end of the day. Usually, Mrs. G gets one arm in the coat and then becomes distracted by something in the environment. She'll then shoot off in the opposite direction, dragging the coat behind her! The staff member usually must follow her, then greet her as if they hadn't been together a few seconds ago: "Hi, Mrs. G. Can I help you with your coat?" If there is another staff person available, one person engages Mrs. G in a conversation while the other helps her get dressed. It takes a few minutes (and a few hundred feet of jogging) to get her ready to go, but it works.

Uncommon Reactions to Common Objects

Mrs. A had been working on a puzzle whose pieces were made of 1/4" thick rubber. She picked up a piece and popped it into her mouth. She took it out a moment later and said, "This meat sure is tough!"

Mrs. S sat down at the table for lunch. On the placemat in front of her were a napkin, fork, glass of milk, and a salad. Mrs. S promptly put the fork into the glass of milk and tried to suck milk through it.

Mrs. M became upset every time that she walked into the bathroom. She apparently became angry at her reflection in the mirror, at which she'd shout and shake her fist.

Mr. L became upset with Mrs. L nearly every evening, sometimes refusing to believe that she was his wife: "You're an old lady! My wife is young! Go away, and bring back my wife!" he'd shout at her. No amount of reassurance or pleading seemed to comfort him.

♪

It's not unusual for persons with dementia to misinterpret common objects or not to recognize people that should be familiar to them. Sometimes, these incidents are easily dealt with (in Mrs. A's case, she spit out the puzzle piece quickly), and sometimes they're devastating (imagine Mrs. L's feelings when her husband of nearly 50 years didn't recognize her).

When a person with dementia reacts in an unusual way to a common object, it's helpful to look at the situation. Sometimes it's possible to understand the mistake and to take measures to prevent such misinterpretations in the future.

Mrs. L was quite upset with Mr. L's inability to recognize her. This usually occurred in the evening, after dinner, when she was in the kitchen cleaning up and Mr. L was sitting in the living room.

At about the same time, Mrs. L noticed that Mr. L was increasingly disturbed by a collection of family photographs that were hung on the living room wall. He was preoccupied with them and would sometimes talk to them. It seemed that it was after he'd been looking at the photos that he became upset with Mrs. L. Several of the photos were of Mr. and Mrs. L when they were quite a bit younger. Mr. L could recognize that they were of himself and his wife, but couldn't make the connection between the young Mrs. L in the photos and the old Mrs. L in the kitchen. When Mrs. L took down the photos from the living room wall, Mr. L's evening outbursts stopped.

Many persons with dementia have unusual reactions to photographs and mirrors. They may become angry at "that guy who's staring at me" or may shout at the mirror's reflection, which is imitating their movements. In such cases, it's helpful to remove or cover the photos or mirrors.

In one of the examples given earlier, Mrs. S mistook her fork for a straw. As she began to have more difficulty recognizing utensils, her place settings were simplified: she was given only her plate and the utensil she needed. Later, the utensils were too difficult for her to use properly so she was served sandwiches and finger foods.

If the person has a great deal of difficulty recognizing objects for what they are, it's helpful to use cuing. (See section on using cues as an aid in communication on page 26.) It's also helpful to look at objects ahead of time, to prepare yourself for any possible misinterpretations:

In grooming class, Mrs. D picked up a hairbrush and began to brush her teeth with it.

Imagine the cooking instructor's surprise when Mrs. E picked up a piece of bread and used it to wipe her nose!

♪

When a person with dementia uses an object in an unusual way, try to redirect him/her in as natural a way as possible. In Mrs. D's case, I may have said, "I can understand why you're using the brush that way, but it works better this way," while demonstrating the proper use of a hairbrush. In Mrs. E's case, I'd probably wait until she was done with the bread, take it away, and then offer her a tissue.

It's important to react calmly to these incidents. The person probably feels embarrassed about using the object in an incorrect way. Try to redirect him/her quietly and discreetly.

I remember reading a story once about a man who was eating in a very high-class restaurant in Hong Kong. He was served a small plate of tiny round objects that resembled candy-coated almonds. He popped one into his mouth and was savoring the delicate crunch of the coating when he looked up and noticed that the woman at the next table was staring at him. She, too, had a plate of the tiny round objects. She peeled hers, as she knew that they were boiled quail eggs.

The point is that all of us have made silly mistakes at one time or another. No one likes to look like a fool. This is important to remember when redirecting the person with dementia who has made a mistake. Point out the mistake kindly and quietly and give assistance and reassurance, just as you would like someone to do for you if you ate a quail egg, shell and all!

Chapter 3

Communication

In a support group for higher-functioning persons with dementia, Mrs. J spoke of the frustration of not being able to communicate clearly: "I don't speak fancy. I speak plain. And sometimes it hurts me when I say something I know ain't right and other people look at me funny. They do this (mimics elbowing another person and rolling her eyes) and it makes me feel real bad."

♪

Communication is perhaps the most frustrating aspect of dementing illnesses, both for the caregiver and the person with dementia. Often, caregivers begin to "give up" and assume that the person doesn't understand what is being said. Caregivers may speak for the person, rather than giving the person a chance to answer for him/herself. Professionals may direct questions to family members or friends, again assuming that the person can't understand what is being said. As the quote above illustrates, this isn't necessarily true. Although the woman in the above example was fairly high-functioning, many lower-functioning people at the AFCC have shown us their ability to understand what is going on around them:

Mrs. B had been a participant in the day center for over two years. By the time she was discharged from the program, she was essentially nonverbal and responded to very little around her. She needed total assistance with her activities of daily living (eating, dressing, personal hygiene) and was unable to walk without assistance. She spent most of the day at the center sitting in a chair staring straight ahead of her, and she no longer appeared to recognize the staff. Her family made the decision to place her in a nursing home, as they were unable to care for her any longer in her deteriorating state. On the day that she was being taken to the nursing home, her daughter noticed tears on Mrs. B's face. She asked, "What's wrong, Mom?" and Mrs. B replied, "I'm going away."

♪

If we were to look at Mrs. B solely on the basis of her needs, it would be clear that she was in the late stage of a dementing illness. It's long been assumed that persons with this level of impairment do not understand what is going on around them. At the AFCC, our experience has been that persons with severe cognitive impairment can comprehend at least some of what is happening to them. The above example illustrates this point. Even though she was very impaired, Mrs. B appeared to understand what was happening to her, and reacted appropriately. It's also interesting to note that Mrs. B, who was essentially nonverbal, managed to so clearly communicate what she was thinking.

The Importance of Nonverbal Communication

Mrs. M watched a staff member walk into the living room of the day center at the end of a long and difficult day. "What's wrong, honey?" she asked. The staff person replied, "Oh, nothing, really. My feet are just tired," not wanting to burden Mrs. M with all of the details of her busy day. Mrs. M looked carefully at the staff member, pointed at her head, and said, "Are you sure you're not tired up here?"

♪

Mrs. M is very confused. She can't remember where she lives or how she gets to and from the day center. She doesn't remember the names of any of the staff or clients that she's with. She's often anxious in the afternoon and will ask again and again, "How am I getting home?" "Do I live here?" "Do you know me?"

For all of her confusion, Mrs. M can read nonverbal communication loud and clear. She can tell immediately if someone is upset or isn't being honest. (She certainly saw through my attempts to hide my feelings from her in the above example.)

Persons with dementia who are unable to understand verbal communication may be able to read nonverbal communication. Often, voice tone and body language are more important than the words that are being spoken:

Mrs. M was sitting with a student in the living room at the day center. She was anxious and asked continually, "How will I get home?" "What time will my husband be here?" and several other questions related to her concerns about getting home. The student patiently answered all of her questions. After a few minutes, with seemingly no provocation, Mrs. M became angry and slapped the student.

♪

The student was answering all of Mrs. M's questions and appeared to be quite patient. Mrs. M didn't key in to his verbal reassurances, though. She noted his exasperation with her through his body language. Before answering yet another round of Mrs. M's questions, he let out a nearly imperceptible sigh. Mrs. M didn't respond to his words, but to this action. (This sigh was truly a tiny one. The only way that we caught it was that this scene was videotaped. We played the scene back several times before we noticed it.)

Body language is particularly important if the person with dementia is anxious or upset. Although you may be taking care to speak softly and calmly, if your body language indicates exasperation, impatience, or anger, this is what the person will react to.

Changed Communication Patterns

Mr. J was trying to say something to the recreation therapist (R.T.) at the day center, but could not get the words out. "Are you hungry?" guessed the R.T. "No," said Mr. J. The R.T. whispered in his ear, "Do you need to use the bathroom?" "No," he said. This went on for a few moments, the R.T. guessing and Mr. J shaking his head in dismay. Finally, Mr. J leaned back in his chair and said, with a look of disgust, "I just can't get it."

Mrs. S became upset at her caregiver, who was trying to help Mrs. S change her dirty clothes. She angrily told her caregiver, "You stop that right now or I'll chew you!"

Mrs. N would repeat the word "yes" over and over again and would answer "yes" to every question she was asked, so it was difficult to know when she meant it. Sometimes, she'd say "yes" when asked if she was hungry, but then wouldn't eat. No one was sure how to find out if Mrs. N really needed something.

♪

The above examples are typical of the sorts of communication patterns you may expect to find in persons with dementia. Mr. J experienced difficulty with *word finding*. He could communicate and had something to say, but simply could not come up with the right word. Mrs. S exhibited *word substitution*. She clearly meant to use the word "bite" instead of "chew." The meaning of the word she used was close to that of the one she meant. Mrs. N used *repetitive phrases*. She'd always answer "yes" to questions because "yes" was one of the few words she could say.

Some persons with dementia make up their own words for things and almost seem to speak their own language. Some ramble on and on, seeming to make absolutely no sense. The question is: How do you communicate with people who have so much trouble making themselves understood?

First of all, it's important for caregivers to listen carefully to everything the person has to say, even if it doesn't seem to make sense at first. Caregivers often discount the communication of persons with dementia only to find that the person was making sense:

Mr. T walked into the kitchen. "When am I going home?" he asked. "Your daughter will pick you up at 3:00, half an hour from now," replied the staff member. "I gotta go home," said Mr. T, "I gotta pay a bill." "Three o'clock is pretty early," the staff person replied. "You'll have plenty of time to pay your bill after you leave here." "You don't understand!" shouted Mr. T. "I gotta pay a water bill!"

♪

If I had looked closer at Mr. T during this exchange, I would have noticed that he was pacing a bit and darting his eyes around the room, looking for something, which turned out to be the bathroom. (I figured this out after he used the word "water.") Who knows? Maybe he always said, "I gotta pay a bill" to excuse himself gracefully. Men of his generation often use phrases like "I gotta see a man about a dog" for this purpose. If I continued to take his words literally, I'd not only have annoyed him, but he'd likely have had an embarrassing accident as well.

Mr. T may have resorted to using the phrase "I gotta pay a bill" because he couldn't think of the word for the bathroom. **Word finding** is a common problem for persons with dementia. The person may be holding a normal conversation, but may then freeze because s/he just can't think of the right word. In this case, it's best to wait a few seconds before suggesting words, as this may destroy the person's train of thought. (Each one of us has been in the situation of trying to remember a name or a piece of information while a well-meaning person cued us so much we forgot our thought completely!) Resist the temptation to suggest words unless (1) you're fairly confident you know what the person means or (2) the person asks for your help or replies positively when you ask if you can suggest words. If the person can't think of the word after a few minutes, you may say to the person, "I'm not sure what you mean. Think about it some more, and if you remember, tell me." In a case like Mr. J's, where he was obviously very frustrated, you may even want to say, "It must be frustrating, not being able to think of the words you need." Acknowledging the person's frustration lets him/her know that you may not understand the words, but you do understand and respect feelings.

Word substitution is similar to word finding, except that the person may use a word that sounds similar to the one intended or to one that is similar in meaning. Here is an example of word substitution: Instead of saying, "I'm looking for my purse," the person says "I'm looking for my verse" or "I'm looking for my suitcase." If you think you know what the person means, you may just want to say, "Your purse? I'll help you find it," rather than correcting the person. In this way, you acknowledge that you know what the person is looking for without embarrassing him/her. If you're not sure of what the person means, you may say, "I'm not sure what you mean. Can you describe it for me?" The person may be able to describe the item or tell you what it's used for, even if s/he can't think of the word for it.

Repetitive phrases are more difficult to work with. In Mrs. N's case, it's obvious that her "yes" answers aren't always reliable. The word "yes" has lost its meaning for her. She uses it because it's one of the few words she has left in her vocabulary. In Mrs. N's case, it's important to look at her body language to determine her true answer. She can still nod and shake her head, and this is a more accurate form of communication than her verbal answers.

Some persons with dementia use repetitive phrases as a form of self-stimulation—the constant repetition of a word or a sound is reassuring or pleasurable to the person. The repetitive phrases may end once the person is engaged in some form of conversation or activity. The person may revert back to using the repetitive phrase during an activity until redirected to the task. Don't assume that the person is unable to communicate reliably just because a repetitive phrase is used:

Mrs. B, a woman with Alzheimer's disease, was a resident in a nursing home. She would sit in a wheelchair in the lounge and say, "Help me, help me" over and over again. She appeared small and frail and looked to be quite confused.

♪

But she wasn't! When I approached Mrs. B, who I'd never met before, I expected that she wouldn't be able to carry on a conversation. Was I wrong! I approached her and asked, "Can I help you?" and she said, "No, I'm all right. Who are you?" We spoke for several minutes. In talking to the aides, and later observing her when her son came to visit, I saw that in addition to her dementia, she was also visually impaired and quite deaf. Her calls of "Help me, help me" may have been self-stimulation, or a prayer.

What do you do when faced with a person whose language is so confused that you can't make any sense out of it? What would you say if a person approached you and said, quite seriously, "The boy he got done now. Yes, he did. I told him, don't give us it. The dogs run away." I've met a number of persons with dementia who are incredibly sociable, warm, and fun to be with, but that communicate in this way. I don't know if there is one right way to communicate with these persons, but I do know of several *wrong* ways:

Ignoring what the person has to say

Laughing at the person's attempts to communicate

Becoming angry at the person's inability to communicate clearly

Talking about the person in front of him/her

Talking down to the person

Mrs. L talks in this way. Her words make little sense, but she is very talkative and friendly. I rarely understand her but sometimes I can pick up on a word or two and carry on a conversation. In answer to the quote mentioned earlier, I might ask, "Did the dogs come back?" or, "That boy sounds like bad news." I may even say, "Mrs. L, I like talking to you. I don't always understand you, but you're fun to talk to."

Mrs. L loves to sing. She mixes up the words to songs just as she does in speech and often comes up with some interesting interpretations of song verses. But we have a great time singing together.

Using Cues as an Aid in Communication

Mr. B. boarded the day center bus and began to walk up and down the aisle, not knowing what he should do. The bus driver noted Mr. B's confusion and gave him a verbal cue: "Please sit down, Mr. B." When this did not work, the driver patted a seat and repeated, "Please sit here," which focused Mr. B on the seat. The staff member then took Mr. B's hand, led him to the seat, and sat on one half of the seat while saying to Mr. B, "Sit down with me." After the staff member demonstrated "sitting down" a few times, Mr. B understood and did so.

♪

If a person with dementia is having difficulty understanding what is expected of him/her, cues may help. There are three different kinds of cues: **Verbal cues** are instructions given to clarify what is expected of the person. Mr. B did not know what to do when he boarded the bus, so the driver gave him a verbal cue: "Please sit down, Mr. B." Mr. B did not respond to the verbal cue, so the driver used a **sensory cue**: patting the seat while repeating the instruction. Finally, a **physical cue** was used: the driver took Mr. B's hand, led him to a seat, and demonstrated what she was asking him to do.

It may not be necessary to use all three kinds of cuing with an individual. Some people may respond well to verbal cues alone or may be able to understand verbal cues accompanied by sensory cues. Only if these two kinds of cuing are used without success, should the caregiver use physical cues. Always assume the person can perform a task with a minimum of cuing. You can always go to the next level of cuing, and this is much easier than smoothing the ruffled feathers of a person whom you've offended.

The following steps may be helpful when using cues:

1. **Establish eye contact.** Make sure that the person you are cuing knows that you are talking to him/her. Look the person directly in the eye and see that s/he is looking you directly in the eye, too. Often caregivers make the mistake of trying to give direction before having the person's attention.

2. **Give a verbal command.** Tell the person what you'd like her/him to do. Keep the direction short and to the point. In Mr. B's case, the direction was, "Please sit here, Mr. B."

3. **Wait a few moments, then try again.** The person with dementia may understand what is being asked but may need a little extra time to respond. Try to avoid giving too many instructions, or repeating instructions too quickly. This will only confuse or frustrate the person. Sometimes it helps to simplify the instructions. For example, if the person with dementia has difficulty understanding the direction, "Have a seat," try "Sit down."

4. **Give a sensory cue.** Again, making sure you have the person's attention, give the direction accompanied by a visual cue. In Mr. B's case, this cue was the patting of the seat the staff member wished him to sit in.

5. **Give a physical cue.** Give the direction while physically indicating what you'd like the person to do. The staff person in Mr. B's example said, "Sit down with me," took Mr. B's hand, and sat down.

6. **Give reassurance and praise.** The person who has difficulty communicating is often embarrassed at his/her inability to understand instructions and may feel badly even after the interaction is completed. A smile, a touch, and verbal reassurance can help the person to feel that you accept him/her, even though the previous interaction may have been difficult: "Thank you, Mr. B. Now we're ready to go home."

If communication problems are difficult for caregivers, realize that they are twice as difficult for the person experiencing them. Be patient, listen carefully to the feelings as well as the words, and be as clear as possible in your communication. Speak slowly and simplify your communication. Don't bombard the person with too many words. Give the person time to respond. Use phrases that are easy to interpret such as, "Sit down" instead of "Have a seat."

Be careful of your voice tone. Sometimes, in our efforts to simplify communication for the person with dementia, we infantilize the person. Don't call the person "sweetie," "honey," "dear," or other terms of endearment unless you've earned the right to use them. Don't use the same tone of voice you would with a child. Use the same tone of voice you'd use with any adult.

It takes practice to learn these techniques. Don't feel bad if at times you still can't understand what the person is saying or can't get the person to understand you. After all, communication is very complex, even with so-called "normal" people.

Humor

Remember to keep your perspective. Having a good sense of humor is helpful when working with or caring for a person with dementia. Many persons with dementia are aware of their deficits and need to talk about them and perhaps joke about them. Mrs. S, a woman that attends the AFCC, likes to say,

"My whole life, I knew I had rocks in my head, but now, the doctors have proved it!"

Just recently, I took a few AFCC participants on a field trip. On the way, I had to put gas in the van. I pulled up to the gas pump, got out of the van, and realized the gas tank was on the opposite side. So, I climbed back in, pulled up to the other side of the pump, and realized I'd done it again. It took me four tries to finally get it right. When I got back in the van, Mrs. S and Mr. G were laughing. Mrs. S noted that the side of the van had the word "Alzheimer's" on it, and that the gas station employees probably thought the van was being driven by "one of 'em!"

The AFCC participants always get a laugh when anyone on the staff misplaces something. I am incapable of going through the morning without losing my coffee cup at least once, which often makes me the butt of the participants' jokes. When I've misplaced something or seem a bit scattered, I'll hear comments from the participants like, "Talk about the blind leading the blind!"

Humor can be used to diffuse difficult situations. On one particularly anxious afternoon when it was difficult to start the group because several participants were asking about going home, I said, "Okay. I've been patient for a while here, but honestly, you guys sound like a broken record! Let's get this out of our systems for once and for all!" We then sang a rousing chorus of "Show Me the Way to Go Home." After this, we had a good laugh and began the activity.

On another day, I'd planned a songwriting group. I began the group with some "bounce" questions, including, "On a scale of one to ten, how do you feel today?" Mr. P said, "Zero. I feel lousy!" (Mr. P *always* says he feels lousy, even when he's smiling and laughing.) So, we wrote a song called "I Feel Lousy," to the tune of "I've Got Sixpence":

I feel lousy, sad and blue.
I feel lousy. Why don't you?
I feel lousy in the morning,
And in the afternoon.
I feel lousy, I don't feel good,
And I don't know why I should!

Now, when Mr. P says he feels lousy, we sing the song together. It always makes him smile.

People with dementia have few chances to really laugh and enjoy themselves. There is certainly a time and a place for serious discussion of feelings. But like anyone else, people with dementia need to have a good time, too.

Chapter 4

Program Development

Mr. S enjoyed attending the music groups offered at the day center. He would sing along with the group leader and had excellent recall for song lyrics, although his verbal communication skills were generally quite poor. His facial expression brightened in music groups and he'd often move in rhythm with the music. Mr. S had the need to pace. Although this was not especially disturbing to the group leader, it was distracting and annoying to the higher-functioning group participants, who would berate Mr. S: "Why don't you sit down? What's the matter with you?" Mr. S also had a tendency to stand directly in front of the group leader, and to try to strum the guitar occasionally while she was playing it, which further upset the other group members.

Mr. C played the harmonica. When he first began attending the day center, he was able to play along with the music group leader in the correct key and rhythm. As his dementia progressed, he found it difficult to keep up but continued to be able to provide a harmonic accompaniment to the music. Eventually he played in an entirely different key and rhythm than the leader did. His diminishing musical ability was disturbing to him, because he could not derive the same pleasure from playing that he once did.

Mrs. R was generally quite restless while at the day center, choosing to sit in on groups but not to participate in most of them. Mrs. R would participate in music groups. She had a strong voice and would occasionally agree to lead songs. After a time, she became anxious in the larger group and was unable to participate in its activities, music included.

♪

Like each of us, persons with dementia are, first and foremost, individuals. Dementia affects each person differently. One person may simply appear forgetful and exhibit no major changes in behavior. Another person may develop the need to pace. Still another may withdraw from social contact altogether, becoming easily overstimulated.

It is easy to see, then, why it is not necessarily good practice to put a group of persons with dementia together for an activity without first taking into consideration the individuals' abilities and needs. As the above examples illustrate, some individuals may need a more structured and supportive environment in order to successfully participate in musical experiences. Their inability to participate in the group at the same level as the others does not mean that the group is not good for them or that they cannot handle music; it simply means that they would respond better to a different approach.

In Mr. S's case, it became apparent to the day center staff that he needed to be in an environment where he could move about freely without receiving negative comments from others. He eventually was placed in a special program at the day center for persons who need to pace. Because everyone in this program had the need to pace, Mr. S's pacing was not disturbing or distracting to the others in the group. Mr. S could then participate in activities in his own way.

Mr. C's case was resolved differently. Recognizing his diminishing ability to play the harmonica, Mr. C's wife began to encourage him to leave his harmonica at home. Mr. C then began to whistle in the music group. He was a terrific whistler and received many compliments from other group participants regarding his talent. As time went on, he began to whistle tunes and rhythms that were unrelated to the music group subject. When his inability to follow the rest of the group interfered with his ability to successfully participate in it, Mr. C was then taken into a quiet room and given a Walkman to listen to. Mr. C looked forward to this time and even went to the public library with his wife to choose tapes to bring to the day center. During his quiet time he would sit in a chair, an intense expression on his face, swaying with the music.

When the group became too stimulating for Mrs. R, she was placed into a smaller music group of four women. She began to actively participate in music again and even sang on a "day center sing-along" tape.

To further illustrate the importance of planning music activities around the clients' remaining abilities, I'd like to describe the evolution of the program at the AFCC. Our observations, combined with the information that we have been offered by AFCC participants and their families, have helped us to develop a supportive model of care for persons with dementia.

Client-Centered Programming for Persons with Dementia

When the AFCC opened in June of 1987, there was little written material on activity programming for persons with dementia. Whenever a book or an article was published on dementia care, we "ate" it up. We corresponded with other dementia programs and visited a few of them. We attended conferences and workshops. And like many dementia-specific programs, we primarily learned what works and what doesn't through trial and error.

In the beginning, our program was run out of a large schoolroom in an old public school building in Chicago that had been bought by a community organization. Our offices and activity area were in the same room. This was a nightmare—imagine trying to run an activity when the telephones are ringing or when visitors walk through the activity area to get to the office. The windows had wire grating over them, left over from the days when the building housed a school and an occasional baseball may have been lobbed at a classroom window. Some of the participants misinterpreted the grating and feared that they were in jail or a concentration camp. The ceilings were high and the floors hardwood, causing sound to echo.

Despite these obvious environmental flaws, the program itself was a success, largely due to a creative, energetic, and determined staff that did everything they could to adapt the environment to the participants' needs. The staff observed the participants carefully and became adept at identifying possible means of overstimulation.

Very early in the AFCC's evolution, it became apparent to staff that there was a need to provide two separate kinds of programming to the participants. The majority of the AFCC's participants were moderately impaired, meaning they were basically independent in their activities of daily living (ADLs) such as feeding, dressing, bathing, and toileting, but may have needed occasional cues. They were able to communicate their needs verbally or through a combination of verbal and nonverbal communication. They were sociable and could tolerate being with groups of 10-12 others without being overstimulated.

The second group of participants was more confused and needed assistance with their ADLs. Many were incontinent. Most were unable to tolerate the stimulation of a large group of people and most were easily distracted. Some were extremely passive and required one-to-one intervention to solicit participation in activities and personal care. Some needed to pace and could not sit down for activities. More than anything else, these persons needed a smaller group and more attention from staff.

The AFCC staff decided to begin programming for two groups. The first group described above was called "The Main Group," as it was the largest group. The second was called "The Sensory Group" because of the participants' lowered tolerance for environmental stress as well as their need for carefully planned sensory stimulation activities.

In December 1988, the AFCC moved into its own building. The new environment was more conducive to client-centered programming since groups could be held in separate rooms and the environment could be controlled in each program area. When we moved into this building, it became possible to further separate the groups. The persons who needed to pace were put into their own group, called "The Walking Club." The AFCC now had three separate programs in one, depending upon the needs of the individual.

In 1990, a fourth group was developed called "The Service Club." This group was designed for persons who are normally a part of the Main Group but who become anxious in the afternoon. This group provided a more structured, intimate environment for clients than did the Main Group.

The AFCC structure is constantly changing, reflecting the changing abilities and needs of the participants. We have given much thought to the ideal program for persons with dementia and have theorized from six to nine potential environments for dementia clients, depending upon their ability to tolerate stimulation and to perform ADLs and on their social interaction and motor skills.

We strongly believe in adapting the environment to meet the needs of persons with dementia. Because of our commitment to this end, our average length of stay has increased from eight months in our first two years to eleven months now in the fourth year of the program. We have had a number of clients participate in our program until just a few months prior to their deaths; a few have died while still participants in the program.

The most significant lessons that we have learned have been from the participants themselves, who are quite vocal about their care preferences and their wish to remain independent for as long as possible. A predominant theme at the AFCC is that of feeling unwanted and useless:

"My daughter-in law does everything for me. I could do things for myself but she says, 'No, no, I'll do it.' So what can I do? I let her do it."

"They [my family] do all my cooking and [lay out my] clothes for me every day. C [my grandson] brings me my food on a tray, [and gives it to me] like an animal, and says, 'Eat, Grandma.' I should be telling him what to do!"

"I feel so stupid sometimes. I try to do things I used to and I forget how."

♪

These examples illustrate the importance to the person with dementia of remaining as independent as possible for as long as possible. At the AFCC, we take care to treat each person with dignity and respect. We strive to create a supportive environment that maximizes the participants' strengths rather than focusing on the person's weaknesses.

In the chapters that follow, music group descriptions will be given for persons in varying stages of dementia, based upon the AFCC's model. Groups will be described for persons who are higher-functioning or in the early/middle stage of dementia (the Main Group); for persons in the middle/late stages of dementia (the Sensory Group); and for persons who need to pace (the Walking Club). Each chapter contains an introduction that describes more clearly the philosophy behind music programming for that particular group. This is by no means an all-inclusive listing of possible music activities for persons with dementia. Be creative. Use your imagination. You'll be surprised what your group (and you) will be able to do.

Part II

Music Groups for Persons with Dementia

Chapter 5

Practical Considerations in Using Music with Older Adults

An Overview of Geriatric Music Therapy Research

Before you begin planning music groups for persons with dementia, it's important to know what the music therapy research tells us about the older adult's musical preferences and ability to hear, process, and understand music. This section will introduce you to some of this research. A summary of the most important points to remember appears at the end of this section.

Older adults tend to prefer the music that was popular when they were young adults (Gibbons, 1977). This means that people currently in their seventies will prefer the music of the mid-1930s to the mid-1940s. People in their eighties will prefer the music of the mid-1920s to the mid-1930s. This is the music that tends to be associated with high school years, a first good job, marriage, children, etc.

This research is generally true for persons born in mainstream American society but may prove untrue for persons born into minority or ethnic cultures. It's important to determine individual musical preferences and to be open to using ethnic music in your groups.

Joseph Moreno (1988) points out that the music in non-Western cultures is often closely related to the religious traditions and cultural values of that society. Additionally, non-Western cultures tend to integrate all of the creative arts in their traditions; music is just a small part of the total ritual. When working with persons of non-Western cultures, you may want to incorporate other creative arts techniques into your music groups; it would be helpful to study the culture to find out more about its traditions.

As we age, our vocal range tends to diminish (Greenwald and Salzberg, 1979). This means that the majority of recorded music and sheet music that is available is simply too high for most older adults to sing. The vocal range that is most comfortable for older adults is from approximately A below middle C to A above middle C. If you're not musical, this basically means that if the music is too high for you to sing, it's *much* too high for an older adult to sing; and if it's comfortable for you to sing, you will probably need to bring it down a bit more to make it comfortable for older adults to sing. It's helpful to have someone with an alto or bass voice lead sing-alongs, as that person will tend to start the song in a better key for the participants. Or, let one of the participants start the song.

As we age, we also tend to lose the ability to discriminate higher-frequency pitches; we hear lower-frequency pitches much more clearly. This condition is well-documented, and is referred to as presbycusis. One study found that older adults spent more time listening to selections with enhanced higher frequencies than did those who listened to normally recorded music (Smith, 1989). This means that if your stereo equipment includes an equalizer, you may want to raise the volume on higher frequencies (above the 3 kHz level). (Note: For hearing loss that is due to nerve damage and for conditions such as Meniere's disease, it may be best to focus on lower-frequency sound, as enhancement of higher-frequency pitches may be ineffective at best, and physically painful at worst.)

Another study found that older adults tended not to compensate for hearing loss by turning up the volume of recorded music. This research indicates that younger adults, who presumably have less hearing loss, tend to listen to music at louder levels than do older adults (Smith, 1988). In terms of leading music groups for older adults, this implies that louder is not necessarily better, and may actually be uncomfortable for hearing-impaired older adults.

Older adults tend to prefer hearing music at slower tempos. Melissa Brotons had older adults listen to the same musical selection played at three different tempos: slow, medium, and fast. She then asked older adult listeners to identify their tempo preferences. They overwhelmingly preferred the slower tempos (Brotons, 1989). This is not to say that older adults only enjoy slow songs; only that they may prefer fast songs to be played at slightly slower tempos. It may also be that singing at slower tempos is easier because the older person can more easily take breaths.

Brotons also studied the accompaniment preferences of older adults. She played the same songs for older adults with five different accompaniment patterns, then asked the older adults to rank them in order of preference. Here are the accompaniments in order of preference:

1. Live Omnichord or autoharp/live vocals
2. Recorded piano accompaniment with block chords/live vocals
3. Recorded guitar accompaniment/live vocals
4. Recorded single-note piano accompaniment/live vocals
5. Recorded combo accompaniment (electronic keyboard that can be set to sound like a full ensemble)/live vocals

In practical terms, this indicates two things: The simpler the accompaniment, the better; and live music is received better than is recorded music.

Reminiscence can be enhanced through musical interventions. In one study, several types of materials were used to elicit reminiscences in elderly nursing home residents. The participants in this study responded better to general questions and historical summaries than to music alone as a means of stimulating reminiscence (Wylie, 1990.) The researcher suggests that using music in conjunction with other conditions may have greater therapeutic benefit than using music alone.

Reigler (1980) compared two kinds of reminiscence formats for disoriented older adults, one with music and one without music. She found that the group that included music as part of the format shared more memories than the group that did not include music.

Much has been written on the positive effect music has on persons with dementia. Millard and Smith (1989) studied the effect of group singing on persons with dementia and found significantly higher vocal/verbal participation among participants during group singing activities. Less wandering and increased interaction between group participants was also noted.

Clair and Bernstein (1990) found that in severely regressed persons with dementia, vibrotactile stimulation (sensory stimulation that involves the sensation of vibrations) was the preferred form of stimulation in music therapy sessions. The participants were offered singing activities, nonvibrotactile instrument playing experiences (hitting a drum held in front of them), and vibrotactile instrument playing experiences (playing a drum held on their lap). The participants overwhelmingly preferred the vibrotactile experience.

This is by no means the be-all and end-all of music therapy research with older adults. But it does give us some practical suggestions for planning groups for older adults:

1. **Music preferences—American popular music.** Focus on the music that was popular when the individual was a young adult.
2. **Music preferences—ethnic music.** Find out as much as you can about the individual's culture and traditions as well as the music itself. Be aware that the music may have religious values or cultural traditions associated with it.
3. **Vocal range of older adults.** Vocal range diminishes as we age; it tends to be strongest at A below middle C to A above middle C.
4. **Changes in the sense of hearing.** As we age, we tend to lose the ability to hear higher frequencies. It is not helpful to turn up the volume to compensate for this kind of hearing loss. Instead, enhance the higher frequencies only; or avoid them altogether and focus on lower frequencies, which are naturally easier for us to hear as we age.
5. **Slow down.** Older adults prefer slightly slower tempos, but not necessarily slower songs.
6. **Accompaniment—simple is best.** Older adults prefer simple chords or one-note accompaniment rather than complex accompaniment.
7. **Music in reminiscence.** Music combined with questions and historical information may help to make reminiscence more effective. Music is an effective tool in increasing participation and orientation of older persons.
8. **Music as sensory stimulation.** Vibrotactile stimulation (sensory stimulation that involves the sensation of vibrations) holds the attention of persons in the late stages of a dementing illness even when other kinds of musical experiences elicit little reaction.

Chapter 6

Music Programming at the Alzheimer's Family Care Center

"The Main Group": Working with Higher-Functioning Persons with Dementia

AFCC participants are placed in the Main Group because of the following strengths and needs:

The Main Group: Strengths

1. The ability to communicate verbally, nonverbally, or through a combination of the two
2. The ability to perform activities of daily living (ADLs) independently or with special set-up/cues
3. The ability to tolerate multisensory stimulation
4. The ability to tolerate groups of 10 persons or more
5. Socially appropriate behavior; recognition of self/others; good-to-fair impulse control (the ability to recognize and control one's own behavior)
6. Ability to tolerate normal changes in the environment (e.g., new people, new activities, etc.)

The Main Group: Needs

1. Activities designed to accommodate the symptoms of distractibility and shortened attention span
2. A closed, distraction-free environment (no extraneous noise, motion, or visual stimulation)
3. A new focus every 15 minutes or so to work with shortened attention spans
4. Emotional support
5. Environmental cues to support independence

Cognitive ability is not necessarily a factor in assigning participants to groups at the AFCC. If a person meets the above criteria, s/he is placed into the Main Group. In fact, the majority of our higher-functioning participants would be considered to be low-functioning in other settings.

To illustrate this, consider that the average Main Group participant scores only an average of 8 points on the Folstein Mini-Mental State Exam. This is a test of general orientation to time, place, and person. A perfect score is 30 points; you or I would probably score 28-30 points (one of the questions is to count backwards from 100 by sevens; I am abysmal with numbers). It is likely, you would not realize at first that the main group participants are as impaired as they are, because their social abilities are largely intact.

Even our highest-functioning participants tend to have shortened attention spans. Because of this, groups are usually planned in 15- or 20-minute segments: several short activities built around one theme. We also go in with more material than we may need for an hour-long session, so that if the participants are unable to participate in one segment of the activity, for whatever reason, the group leader can switch to another idea.

General Goals

The Main Group participants are generally aware that there is something wrong with their memory, even if they cannot always articulate their diagnosis. Since our day center is named "The Alzheimer's Family Care Center," it would be difficult for us to keep the cause of the participants' memory problems from them for very long. Although all participants do not have a diagnosis of Alzheimer's disease, every participant has been diagnosed with some form of chronic, irreversible dementia. (See the section "A Brief Overview of Alzheimer's Disease and Related Dementias," page 7.)

Several of our Main Group participants are members of a client support group that focuses on issues of importance to persons with dementia. Since I am a co-leader of this group, the themes discussed help me, in turn, to plan groups that can focus on the clients' issues. Some of the predominant themes thus far have been:

- Loss of independence/autonomy
- Fear of getting lost
- Fear of "losing your mind"
- Disrespect from family members, professionals
- Feeling misunderstood
- Feeling lonely
- Depression

Working with these common feelings, music is used in the Main Group at the AFCC to:

1. Provide the opportunity for autonomy and decision making (participants are encouraged to bring in their own favorite music or to give suggestions for future music groups)
2. Give participants the opportunity to voice their opinions
3. Provide the opportunity to discuss feelings in a supportive, accepting environment
4. Increase self-esteem and enhance sense of self through memories of past accomplishments, significant others, and significant life events
5. Assess and maintain eye/hand coordination, fine- and gross-motor coordination, reading skills, recognition of common

objects, ability to follow complex directions (more than one step)

6. Provide a means of creative self-expression
7. Provide a means of nonverbal communication
8. Elicit extramusical associations (memories)
9. Most importantly, have fun!

Chapter 7

Adapting Music Groups

It is possible to do nearly the same music activities with higher-functioning persons with dementia that you do with any group of cognitively-intact older adults, with a few adaptations:

1. **Simplify instructions.** Don't give all of the instructions for an activity at once. Give them one at a time and make sure the first step is understood before giving the next step.

2. **Slow down and be patient.** Persons with dementia need more time to process information than do persons with no cognitive deficits. You can help by slowing down and giving additional cues when the person seems to need them.

3. **Avoid open-ended questions.** The person with dementia may have difficulty answering a question such as "How do you feel about...?", but may be able to answer the question "Does it make you angry when...?" You'll get more accurate answers if you ask questions that require specific answers.

4. **Concentrate on long-term memories.** Persons with dementia tend to have better long-term than short-term memory.

5. **Encourage participation, right or wrong.** Persons with dementia are constantly reminded of what they can't do. If a participant gives a wrong answer to a question, don't discourage him/her; thank him/her for trying, or give additional cues to help find the correct answer.

6. **Don't be afraid to try new things.** Persons with dementia need variety just as much as you and I do. Take a risk. Try something new and unusual in your sessions. If it doesn't work, then you can always go back to a familiar activity.

The participants and I decided to try organizing a bell choir at the AFCC. I expected it to be a bit difficult for even the higher-functioning group, but they proved me wrong. Although I've had to make a few adaptations to accommodate individual participants' needs, it continues to be a positive activity for the group. If the participants and I were afraid to try new things, we'd never have started a bell choir.

For additional books and materials that can be adapted for use with higher-functioning persons with dementia, see the Appendix.

Chapter 8

Reminiscence Groups

It is comforting to persons with dementia to remember the "good old days" before their memory was impaired. Reminiscence is a way for them to tell others what their lives were like before the dementia changed everything. Reminiscence can also help the person with dementia keep in touch with his/her past and to maintain a sense of identity.

Robert Butler discussed the phenomenon of reminiscence as a natural, integral process of aging, and he believed that it should be encouraged whenever possible. He felt that reminiscence could be used towards therapeutic ends, as well as for its own sake, by helping the older adult to resolve past conflicts and find meaning in his/her life. He termed this therapeutic reminiscence "Life Review," and outlined a detailed assessment and treatment process to help evoke crucial memories in the individual (Butler, 1963; Butler and Lewis, 1982).

Reminiscence groups are particularly important for the person with dementia, who may not be able to reminisce independently. Stimulating long-term memory can have a positive effect on the person who sees himself/herself only as s/he is now.

The groups described in this section do not constitute a Life Review Therapy program, but can certainly be used to elicit reminiscence in a therapeutic way.

It's important to note that negative, as well as positive, memories may surface during these sessions. The group leader must be prepared to deal with these feelings. For example, a reminiscence group on the topic of babies or children may bring back memories of a child who died in infancy or feelings of sadness in a person who never had children. It is not necessary to exclude persons with these feelings from the session; if handled properly, these memories may help the person come to grips with a negative experience.

Tearful reactions to music and memories are not uncommon and are not always negative. I personally get teary-eyed whenever I hear a drum cadence; it reminds me of the great times I had as a member of my high school marching band. Don't overreact to tears; but do pay attention to them.

Above all, listen to the participants because one group can lead to another. Perhaps, while reminiscing on the topic of school, someone will remember the old Palmer method of penmanship, which stimulates memories of other learning experiences. This may then be used as a topic for the next reminiscence session. Look for local attractions or experiences that the participants may enjoy reminiscing about. For example, two sure-fire Chicago hits are Riverview Park (a Chicago amusement park that closed in 1967—I was never there, but can I tell you stories!) and the Century of Progress Exposition, held in Chicago from 1933-1934.

You'll notice that the following six reminiscence groups rely heavily on props and prompts from the group leader. Persons with dementia don't always respond well to open-ended questions such as, "Who was your favorite singer?" Closed questions work better: "Did you like Bing Crosby? How about Frank Sinatra?"

These groups strive to elicit reminiscences by stimulating all of the senses: vision, hearing, touch, smell, and taste. As such, they are sensory stimulation groups as well as reminiscence groups.

When leading these reminiscence groups, it's a good idea to have a blackboard, whiteboard, or flip chart available to write down interesting or significant reminiscences. At the AFCC, we recently reminisced on the topic of "occupations" and I made a list of the participants' memories of their first job. We left the list up all day, and staff and families enjoyed reading what kinds of jobs people had held. The list encouraged staff and families to reminisce about their first jobs and elicited further reminiscing in the persons who had participated in the group. Staff also had a new perspective on the participants ("John worked as a shoemaker? That explains why he was admiring my shoes the other day!"). You know a group has had an impact if it can touch so many people.

Several times participants in AFCC groups have shared memories that sounded implausible but were actually true, like the peppermint-stick-in-a-pickle story mentioned in the "Toyland" group. When in doubt, ask if anyone else remembers a similar memory, because often, someone will.

The bibliography and resource list in this book contain several resources for reminiscence group plans and nostalgia. Often, the best resource for nostalgia is garage or rummage sales. I once bought a whole box of sheet music dating back to the 1920s and 1930s, in excellent condition, for only $5.00 at a church rummage sale.

One more note: Although I suggest using songsheets in the following groups, I'm aware that not all persons with dementia are able to use them successfully. Use your judgment. You may want to write the lyrics out on a large sheet of paper that gets posted on a board in the room if songsheets are too distracting.

These are the goals for the following music and reminiscence groups:

1. Opportunity for choice
2. Opportunity to voice opinions
3. Opportunity to discuss feelings
4. Opportunity for autonomy and decision making
5. Elicit reminiscences through extramusical associations
6. Increase self-esteem and sense of self through memories of past accomplishments, significant others, and significant life events
7. Elicit reminiscences through sensory stimulation

"You Must Have Been a Beautiful Baby"

Group Preparation

A few weeks before presenting this session, begin collecting photos or drawings of babies. You can do this as an arts and crafts project and create a collage of baby pictures from magazines.

If possible, contact participants and their caregivers or families about bringing in their baby pictures, or pictures of their children or grandchildren as babies. This is more easily done in a community-based setting or in the home than in a long-term care setting, but adds much to the quality of the session. Also, bring in your baby pictures and approach other staff about bringing in theirs. As you receive baby photos, post them on a bulletin board with the message: "You must have been a beautiful baby...can you tell who is who?" with a list of names and perhaps current photos of these persons.

Props

- rattles
- diaper pins
- small stuffed animals
- bottles
- teething rings
- jars of baby food
- diapers (cloth and disposable)
- receiving blankets
- baby lotion, powder
- at least one musical toy, preferably one that plays a familiar childhood tune such as Brahms' lullaby or "Twinkle, Twinkle, Little Star"

Suggested Songs

"Twinkle, Twinkle, Little Star"
"Lullaby and Goodnight" (Brahms' lullaby)
"Hush, Little Baby"

Group Procedure

Set-up. Chairs in a semi-circle, facing the bulletin board with the photos (or the collage), and a small table with the props on it. You will also want a blackboard, white board, or flip chart. You'll need a tape player, phonograph, or CD player (if you choose to use recorded music).

Setting the mood. As participants arrive, allow them to examine the photos and the baby items. Play a recording of lullabies, music box music, or childhood songs while people are getting settled.

Opening song. "You Must Have Been a Beautiful Baby"

Topic introduction. *"We may not remember much about what it was like to be a baby, but almost every one of us has had experience with babies. We may have helped with our younger brothers or sisters, babysat when younger, raised children or grandchildren of our own, or assisted family or friends with their children."*

Visual stimulation. Show the baby photos. If you received photos of staff or participants, match the photo with the person.

Intellectual stimulation. Have participants name everything they can think of that babies need. Make a list on the board. It may help to try to think of one item for every letter of the alphabet:

A - A & D ointment (for diaper rash)
B - bassinet
C - crib, cradle
D - diapers, etc.

Props/tactile stimulation. Pass around the baby items. Have participants tell what the items are, how they are used, and encourage reminiscing about them.

Smell/taste stimulation. Encourage participants to put a bit of baby oil, powder, or lotion on their hands. The tactile and olfactory stimulation may elicit memories. You may even want to ask if anyone would be willing to taste a bit of baby food, to see what s/he thinks of it. If you're going to do this, try a pleasant-tasting flavor like chocolate pudding or bananas, not strained carrots! For the ultimate in sensory stimulation, see if anyone on the staff would be willing to bring in his/her infant or toddler for the participants to visit with and, possibly, to hold.

Music/singing. Hand out songsheets and sing the lullabies. This would be especially appropriate if a baby is present. If not, ask about putting a baby to sleep: *"Did you ever sing a lullaby to calm a baby? Did the singing work? Why or why not?"* Also, share the musical toys. *"Did you have any musical toys when you were a child, or did you have any for your children or grandchildren? Did you/the children like them? Do you remember what the toy looked like?"*

Closure. To close, thank everyone for coming and sharing their memories. Close with a goodbye song (the AFCC's current favorite is "Till We Meet Again"). If possible, hand out a souvenir or novelty, such as a baby shower favor, as a reminder of the group.

Additional Suggestions

I brought my baby album to a group, along with a pair of baby shoes. The shoes were a big hit because they were real—I'd worn them when I was a baby. They were obviously old and beat up and were reminders of the baby shoes of over thirty years ago.

You may want to ask the participants to give new parents some advice. *"What would you tell a set of new parents, in light of what you've learned over the years?"*

You may want to ask the women what they remember about being pregnant and about having the baby. Things were much different back then. Few fathers were able to see their children being born; you may want to ask the men what it felt like to be in the waiting room.

"Toyland"

Group Preparation

The focus of this group is children's songs that are often associated with children's games. Before the group, you may consider making a collage of school-age children (which would also be appropriate for the next group in the series), collecting photos of participants and staff as school-age children, and developing a photo-board (as described for the previous group).

Props

- marbles
- playground balls
- jacks
- a baseball and bat
- jump ropes
- a catcher's mitt
- a rag doll
- a yo-yo
- a slingshot
- a Mother Goose book
- peppermint sticks
- bubblegum
- sidewalk chalk (for drawing hopscotch squares)

Suggested Songs

"London Bridge"
"Mary Had a Little Lamb"
"Little Sally Saucer"
"Twinkle, Twinkle, Little Star"
"Ring Around the Rosies"
"Bingo"

Group Procedure

Set-up. Same as first group, page 44.

Setting the mood. As participants arrive, have recorded children's music playing, such as the "Wee Sing," Mister Rogers, Raffi, or Sesame Street albums.

Opening song. "Toyland." If appropriate, hand out songsheets with the lyrics.

Introduce the topic. *"Today, we're here to talk about what it's like to be a child and, in particular, the kinds of games that children like to play."*

Visual stimulation. Show the group the photos and discuss them. Memory questions: *"Look at how children dressed then compared to now. What's different?"* (Today, girls can wear pants. Young boys wear long pants now, whereas they wore short pants in the 1920s through 1940s. Today, no dress codes in school; jeans are the norm.) *"What did you do for fun when you were a child? What kinds of chores did you have to do at home?"*

Intellectual stimulation. Make a list of games, toys, and things children like:

A - apples (for the teacher, of course!)
B - baseball
C - candy
D - dogs ("Mommy, he followed me home. Can I keep him?")
E - electric trains, etc.

Props/tactile stimulation. Pass around the props. Have the participants examine and discuss them: *"What is this? How did you play with it? Did you have one? Describe it."*

Smell/taste stimulation. Offer each participant a piece of bubblegum or a peppermint stick. (Note: Use sugar-free candy and gum that won't stick to dentures.) You may want to have a bubble-blowing contest. (Several AFCC folks have told me it was a big treat when they were young to put a peppermint stick into a pickle and eat them together. This sounds awful to me, but so many folks have mentioned it that it must have been at least a local tradition.)

Music/singing. Pass out the songsheets and sing the children's songs. If a game is associated with the song, ask the participants how the game was played.

Closure. Thank the participants for coming to the group and sharing their memories, then sing a goodbye song. Keeping with the theme, "Goodnight Ladies" or "Buffalo Gals" may be appropriate.

There's a huge difference in the childhood experiences of rural vs. urban children. This makes for fun exchanges in reminiscence groups. While the urban folks discuss playing mumblety-peg and buck-buck, I can recall teasing bulls to see if we could get them to charge us and "summer sledding" down the banks of a creek on a cardboard box. Some of my rural childhood counterparts can remember similar experiences and more—being chased from the hen house by an angry rooster ("That rooster had the devil in him!" said Mrs. J), and trying to shoot a rabbit for the first time:

"I saw a rabbit from the porch and I thought, if I shoot him, we could eat him for dinner. So I went in the house and I got the shotgun and I aimed, and I was way over to the left. That rabbit just set there and looked at me! So I tried again and I shot in front of the rabbit. He didn't even run, he just set there. I felt so ashamed I run inside and put the shotgun away, and since that day I left the shootin' to the men."

"School Days"

Group Preparation

Gather photos of school children, schools, teachers, etc., for use during the discussion.

Props

- school books
- apples
- large pencils
- a book strap
- fountain pens
- a ruler
- ink bottles
- flash cards
- wide-lined paper
- a chalkboard or slate
- an eraser
- a lunch box or paper bag
- a lard bucket (Seniors who grew up in rural areas may have used an old lard bucket for a lunch pail.)

Smell/Taste Stimulation

Share some penny candy with the group: Maryjanes, root beer barrels, licorice whips, candy buttons (the "dots" on sheets of paper), lollipops, peppermint sticks, caramel bulls-eyes, or Cracker Jacks.

Suggested Songs

Make two sets of songsheets for the group, one of patriotic songs and one of children's songs. Examples:

"America the Beautiful"
"My Country, 'Tis of Thee"
"The National Anthem"
"Yankee Doodle"

"London Bridge"
"Ring Around the Rosies"
"The Alphabet Song"
"Mary Had a Little Lamb"

Group Procedure

Set-up. Same as for first group, page 44.

Setting the mood. As participants enter the room, have recorded music playing that focuses on learning or school, such as Sesame Street tapes or recordings of children singing. Allow participants to look at the props and discuss them.

Opening song. "School Days"

Topic introduction. *"Today's topic is school. Let's try to think about things we liked and disliked about school, both as children and parents. If any of you are former teachers, you can help us to understand what it was like teaching children."*

Visual stimulation. Pass around the photos of children and discuss them: *"Is this how you looked when you went to school? How did you dress? How did you wear your hair? How did you get to school? Did you walk or take a bus? Do you remember any of your teachers? What was the name of your school?"*

Intellectual stimulation. Ask participants to remember how their school day started. For most of the country, it began with the Pledge of Allegiance, a patriotic song, and perhaps a prayer. Recite the Pledge of Allegiance with the group. You'll want to have a flag to face, and you may need to remind people to place their right hand over their hearts.

It's not unusual for older adults to omit the phrase "under God" in the pledge. That's because this phrase was added to the pledge later, after most older adults had already finished grammar school.

Sing the patriotic songs. Perhaps someone in your group will remember singing a different song to begin the day, particularly if s/he attended a religious school. If the person feels comfortable, ask him/her to sing the song for the group. (I've learned lots of songs this way.)

Props/tactile stimulation. Pass around and discuss the props: *"What is this? What was it used for? Do you remember this?"* Begin with the usual school-related items, and end with the graduation items. Ask: *"Who here was lucky enough to graduate from grammar school? High school? College? Who wasn't able to graduate, and why?"*

Smell/taste stimulation. Bring out the penny candy and the apples and let people hold, smell, and taste them (if their diet allows it). Questions: *"Where did you buy penny candy? Can you remember any other kinds? Where did you get the money? Did you ever give a teacher an apple?"*

Music/singing. "Now we're going to talk about everybody's favorite topic—recess!" Sing "London Bridge" and "Ring Around the Rosies." Discuss recess and games played at recess. *"What games did you play? Do you remember the rules?"*

Closure. Thank everyone for participating and sharing their memories. Sing a closing song like "The More We Get Together" (to the tune of "Ach du Lieber Augustine"):

The more we get together,
together, together,
The more we get together,
the happier we'll be.
For your friends are my friends,
and my friends are your friends.
The more we get together,
the happier we'll be.

Additional Suggestions

The subject of school days is so big, you may want to break it up into two groups. There are a number of other possibilities for activities/ discussions:

- A spelling bee
- An "arithmetic lesson" (working with the flash cards)
- Discussion of punishments for misbehaving (like the hickory switch, having your knuckles rapped, standing in the corner, putting your gum on your nose)
- Discussion of "the teacher's pet," "the dunce," and "the class clown"

Occupations

Group Preparation

Perhaps as an arts and crafts group, make a collage of people at work. If you don't have time to do this, or have trouble finding appropriate photos, many teachers' stores carry photo packets of people at work.

Props

- a lunch bucket
- a typewriter ribbon
- a social security card
- a file folder
- a paycheck stub
- a desk calendar
- a train ticket, bus token, or bus pass
- a time card
- any hats that are associated with an occupation, such as a hard hat, a football helmet, a nurse's cap, a fireman's hat, etc.

Smell/Taste Stimulation

Serve coffee or tea and donuts or coffee cake.

Suggested Songs

"Oh, How I Hate to Get Up in the Morning"
"Whistle While You Work"
"I've Been Working on the Railroad"
"Sixteen Tons"
"Heigh-Ho"

Group Procedure

Set-up. Same as for first group, page 44.

Setting the mood. As people enter the room, you may want to play recorded "elevator music" (like Montovani) as this music is often played in offices/factories. Or, if your group would like it, you may want to use a recording of "Nine to Five."

Opening song. "Heigh-Ho" from the film *Snow White*. (This song is especially good because if people don't know the words, they can whistle the tune, just as the dwarfs did.)

Topic introduction. *"Today, we're going to talk about work: What kinds of work we've done and what we thought about it. I'm interested in hearing about not only your favorite jobs, but also the ones you didn't like."*

Visual stimulation. Examine the photos of people at work and discuss them: *"What kind of work is being done in this picture? Have you ever done that? What did you think about it? Have you ever wanted to do that? Does it look like the person in the picture likes what s/he is doing?"*

Intellectual stimulation. Make a list of as many occupations as the group can think of. You may want to come up with one occupation for every letter of the alphabet:

A - army officer
B - baker
C - cook
D - dog breeder/trainer
E - electrician
F - fireman, etc.

After this list is done, start another list of jobs that have been held by people in the room. (Doing the alphabet list first can help to stimulate memory.) For additional cues, ask: *"Do you remember your first job? What was your favorite job? What was the worst job you ever had? What job did you retire from?"*

If there are women in the group who never worked outside of their homes, treat the categories "housewife" or "mother" in the same way you do the others. For example, every housewife has a job she hates. In this way, the women who never held a job outside of the home won't feel excluded.

Props/tactile stimulation. Show the props and discuss them: *"What is this? Did you use it in your work? What is it used for?"*

Smell/taste stimulation. *"It's time for a coffee break."* Serve the coffee/tea and donuts/ coffee cake and reminisce about coffee breaks (or coffee klatsches): *"What kinds of things did you talk about? Who did you take your breaks with? How long were your breaks? How many breaks did you get?"*

Music/singing. Sing the songs and discuss them. For "Oh, How I Hate to Get Up in the Morning": *"What time did you get up? What did you do to get ready for work? How did you get to work?"* Sing and discuss the rest of the songs.

Closure. Thank everyone for coming to the session and for sharing their memories. Sing a closing song such as "Till We Meet Again" or "The More We Get Together."

Additional Suggestions

If you know of any special work-related accomplishments of persons in the group, find out beforehand if they would like to share this information with the group or if they would mind if you do. For example, the AFCC once had a former football star as a participant and he was very happy to bring in his scrapbook and share his accomplishments with the group.

Growing Up

Note: There may be people in the group who have never been married, who are widowed, or who have had, or are still involved in, unhappy marriages. Marriage can be a thorny subject to discuss, so the focus of this session is not simply marriage, but "growing up"—taking responsibility for one's self and becoming independent. For the majority of people, this begins with marriage; so, the first part of this session focuses on weddings and marriage, but it later moves on to topics of adulthood in general.

Group Preparation

Clip photos of brides and weddings, houses, men and women in military uniforms, college graduations or colleges, people at work, parents and children, and any other photos that fit the topic of "adulthood." If possible, bring in a personal wedding photo album, graduation photos, or photos of children for the participants to look at. These latter photos should be of you or someone in the group.

Props

- a wedding invitation
- the deed to a house
- a bridal veil
- a real estate listing
- champagne glasses
- the want ads
- a marriage license
- diapers
- a report card
- utility bills

Note: Not everyone was married in a religious ceremony. Many couples were married in civil ceremonies during WWII when they'd marry quickly before the groom went off to war. In some cases, couples were married twice; once in a civil ceremony before the groom went off to war and a second time in a religious ceremony upon the groom's return.

Couples who married during the Depression and couples that lived in rural areas often had simple receptions, held at the home of the bride's or groom's parents. With the exception of the upper classes, the tradition of formal receptions is a fairly new one.

Suggested Songs

"I'll Be with You in Apple Blossom Time"
"I Love You Truly"
"Let Me Call You Sweetheart"
"There's No Place Like Home"
"Brother, Can You Spare a Dime?"
"Sonny Boy"
"Love Nest"

Group Procedure

Set-up. Same as for first group, page 44.

Setting the mood. As people enter the room, play recorded music from when the participants were young adults, such as big band music or songs popular during WWII.

Opening song. "I Won't Grow Up" from the musical *Peter Pan*. This song looks at growing up from a child's perspective ("for growing up is awfuler than all the awful things there ever were!"), and is a good place to start the discussion.

Topic introduction. *"Today we're going to look at growing up, or becoming an adult. Thinking back, can you remember what it was that made you feel grown up? When did you know you weren't a kid anymore?"*

Visual stimulation. After the discussion, show the photo collage and any personal photos you may have received from the group. Discuss the events depicted in the photos.

Intellectual stimulation. A history quiz:

1. Which president was a Rough Rider and had a cuddly toy named after him later? **Answer:** Teddy Roosevelt (Teddy bear)
2. What important event occurred on Oct. 29, 1929? **Answer:** The stock market crash, which heralded the beginning of the Great Depression
3. What was a flapper? **Answer:** A young society woman of the 1920s; she wore bobbed hair, short dresses (to the knee), long beads, hose rolled down below the knee; she put on her lipstick in such a way to produce the look of "bee stung lips"
4. What were the "Charleston" and the "Black Bottom"? **Answer:** Dances
5. What happened on December 7, 1941? **Answer:** Japanese bombed Pearl Harbor
6. What president, who succeeded FDR, had a sign on his desk that said "The buck stops here"? **Answer:** Harry S. Truman
7. What U.S. president was the only man to be elected to four consecutive terms in office? **Answer:** Franklin D. Roosevelt
8. Whose presidential campaign buttons read, "I like Ike." **Answer:** Dwight Eisenhower
9. What famous 1920s gangster was known as "Scarface"? **Answer:** Al Capone

Props/tactile stimulation. Show the props to the group and discuss them. Wedding items: *"Have you seen these items at a wedding? What are they for? What do you remember about weddings, or about being in love for the first time? Can you remember where you went for your first date?"* Other items: discuss important life events such as graduation, buying a first home, trying to find a good job, or having children. *"What was difficult about these times? What was good? If you had it all to do over again, is there anything you would change?"*

Smell/taste: If possible, serve a cake and coffee to the group. Many of the events we associate with adulthood are celebrated with parties in which the centerpiece is a cake. Decorate the cake with the word, "Congratulations." Ask these questions: "Looking over your lives, what things are you the proudest of? What things do you feel you have done well?" You may want to write these things down on the blackboard for everyone to see.

Music/singing. Sing songs appropriate to the topic and discuss them. Discuss love and commitment with the songs "I'll Be with You in Apple Blossom Time," "I Love You Truly," and "Let Me Call You Sweetheart." Discuss what makes a house (or an apartment) a home with "Love Nest" and "Home Sweet Home." Discuss children and how being a parent changes your life with "Sonny Boy." For "Brother, Can You Spare a Dime?" you could ask, *"Have you ever been out of work? What was that like?"*

Closure. Thank everyone for participating and sharing their memories.

"Sentimental Journey"

Group Preparation

Use the collage from the "School Days" group for this session. In addition, ask group participants or their families to bring in photos of their children and grandchildren for this group.

Props

- a report card
- a 78-rpm record
- a 45-rpm record
- a 33-rpm record
- a cassette tape
- a compact disc
- car keys

Photos of singing stars:

- Al Jolson
- Nat King Cole
- Rudy Vallee
- Connie Francis
- Bing Crosby
- Perry Como
- Frank Sinatra
- Rosemary Clooney
- Ella Fitzgerald
- Andy Williams
- Kate Smith
- Doris Day
- Lena Horne
- Elvis Presley
- Louis Armstrong
- The Beatles

This group focuses on generational differences in music. Be aware that you may have quite an age span in your group, so that a song that was popular when one participant was young may have been the favorite song of another participant's parents.

You may want to use original recorded music for this session. Some suggestions:

"Mammy" or "April Showers" by Al Jolson

"The Whiffenpoof Song" by Rudy Vallee

"The Flat Foot Floogie" by Benny Goodman and his orchestra

"A-Tisket, A-Tasket" by Ella Fitzgerald

"Chattanooga Choo Choo" by Glenn Miller and his orchestra

"Tennessee Waltz" by Patti Page

"Que Será, Será" by Doris Day

"Moon River" by Andy Williams

"(You Ain't Nothin' But a) Hound Dog" by Elvis Presley

"My Generation" by The Who

"I Wanna Hold Your Hand" by The Beatles

If you're feeling adventuresome, you may want to include a rap piece, such as "Ice, Ice Baby" by Vanilla Ice, at the end, so that the group can share their opinions of today's musical trends.

If you decide to use recorded music, adjust the recordings to fit the participants' shortened attention spans or you'll lose their concentration. Use only one or two songs per era, and only short segments of the songs, maybe 30 - 60 seconds.

Group Procedure

Set up. Same as for first group, page 44.

Setting the mood. Have a recording of the song "Kids" (from the musical *Bye, Bye, Birdie*) playing while the participants enter the room. The words to this song are perfect for the group topic, so you may want to have them written down for the participants to look at while the song is playing. Put the props out for the participants to examine.

Opening song. Sing a few songs from the Gay Nineties, such as "After the Ball" or "The Band Played On."

Topic introduction. *"Today, we're going to look at the differences between the generations and at the music in particular. The songs we just sang were probably popular in your parents' or grandparents' time. There was a different kind of popular music in their day, in your day, in your children's day, and today."* Play "Mammy," "April Showers," or "The Whiffenpoof Song" as examples of the music popular in the 1910's and 1920's. Then play "The Flat Foot Floogie" and "A-Tisket, A-Tasket" and discuss the difference in the musical styles. *"Which style do you like best? Why?"*

Visual stimulation. Show the photos, one at a time, and ask the participants to identify the persons in the photos. Ask: *"What did you think about this person? Did you enjoy their music?"*

Intellectual stimulation. A musical quiz:

1. Who is "Ol' Blue Eyes"? **Answer**: Frank Sinatra

2. Who was known as "The Songbird of the South"? **Answer**: Kate Smith

3. Who was known as "The Crooner"? **Answer**: Bing Crosby or Rudy Vallee

4. Who was known as "The Waltz King"? **Answer**: Wayne King

5. Who coined the term "champagne music" to describe his orchestra's sound? **Answer**: Lawrence Welk

6. Whose orchestra was called "The Royal Canadians"? **Answer**: Guy Lombardo

7. This female singer is known for singing the song, "Stormy Weather." **Answer**: Lena Horne

8. What were the Dorsey Brothers' first names? **Answer**: Tommy and Jimmy

9. With what band did Frank Sinatra get his start? **Answer**: Tommy Dorsey's

10. What instrument is nicknamed the "bone"? **Answer**: Trombone

Props/tactile stimulation. Pass around the props and discuss them. For the report card and car keys, you may want to ask if these items ever caused problems in the house. *"Did your kids ever get bad grades? Did they ever want the car on Saturday night? Did your kids get an allowance? What did they have to do to earn it? Did you get an allowance when you were young?"*

Show the records, tapes, and the compact disc. Talk about the difference in not only the music over the past forty or fifty years, but in how it is recorded.

Smell/taste stimulation. Over the last fifty or so years, one tradition has remained constant: going out for a cola, burger, and fries or an ice cream soda. Serve cola and French fries or small hamburgers, if possible. Discuss this: *"Where did you go for a snack with your friends? Do you remember how much a hamburger or an ice cream soda cost back then?"*

Music/singing. Play the recordings for the group, starting with one or two selections from the mid-1920s to mid-1930s, then moving on to music of the 1940s and 1950s. When their music is playing, participants may share memories of going dancing or of meeting members of the opposite sex. When the 1950s and 1960s music is playing, ask: *"What do you think of this? Did you like it when it first came out? Did you ever dance to this? Did your kids/grandkids like this music?"*

If you have photos of the recording artists, it may help to elicit further discussion. Show the photo to the group while the music is playing.

Closure. Sing "Sentimental Journey." Thank everyone for coming and sharing their memories and opinions about music.

Chapter 9

Music Games

The following games are tried-and-true favorites at the AFCC. The beauty of them is that they are noncompetitive in nature and encourage the group members to help one another. Persons with dementia spend so much time being reminded of what they cannot do. Who wants to play a game that is competitive and that you might lose? Nobody loses these games and we have a lot of fun.

General Goals

1. Encourage teamwork
2. Increase self-esteem through opportunity for positive experience
3. Increase verbalization through singing and recitation of rhythmic verse
4. Maintain long-term memory retrieval skills
5. Maintain attending skills
6. For active music games: Provide opportunity for physical exercise; maintain fine- and gross-motor coordination

Complete the Line

The procedure for this game is simple. The leader sings the first few words of a song and the group completes the line. If your group is musical, they may finish the whole song. The leader can sing or speak the words, but singing them is the most effective.

1. "I'll be lovin' you...always"
2. "In the good old...summertime"
3. "Daisy, Daisy...give me your answer, do"
4. "When the red, red, robin...comes bob, bob, bobbin' along"
5. "Let me call you...sweetheart"
6. "Five foot two...eyes of blue"
7. "Oh, give me a home...where the buffalo roam"
8. "You are my...sunshine"
9. "East side, west side...all around the town"
10. "Show me the way to go...home"
11. "Irene...goodnight"
12. "I've been workin' on the...railroad"
13. "How much is that...doggie in the window"
14. "My wild...Irish Rose"
15. "Should old acquaintance...be forgot"
16. "There's a yellow rose in...Texas"

17. "I love you...truly"
18. "Put on your old...grey bonnet"
19. "When Irish eyes...are smiling"
20. "Mairzy doats and...doazy doats"
21. "The flat foot floogie...with the floy floy"
22. "He's got the whole world...in His hands"
23. "She'll be coming 'round the mountain...when she comes"
24. "I'll be seeing you...in all the old familiar places"
25. "When you wore a...tulip"
26. "Don't sit under the apple tree...with anyone else but me"
27. "Casey would waltz with the...strawberry blonde"
28. "After the ball is...over"
29. "Yes, we have no...bananas"
30. "Barney Google...with the goo-goo-googly eyes"
31. "Yes, sir...that's my baby"
32. "Ma, he's making...eyes at me"
33. "Ain't she...sweet"
34. "Way down upon the...Swanee River"
35. "Is it true what they say about...Dixie"
36. "The stars at night are big and bright...deep in the heart of Texas"
37. "Embrace me, my sweet...embraceable you"
38. "Pardon me, boy...is that the Chattanooga choo choo"
39. "Amazing grace...how sweet the sound"
40. "Gonna take a...sentimental journey"
41. "You push the first valve down, the music goes around and around, oh...and it comes out here"
42. "Oh, the sun shines bright...on my old Kentucky home"
43. "Take me out to the...ball game"
44. "School days, school days...dear old golden rule days"
45. "I'll take you home again...Kathleen"
46. "The hills are alive...with the sound of music"
47. "Chicago, Chicago...that toddlin' town"
48. "I left my heart...in San Francisco"
49. "Meet me in St. Louis, Louis...meet me at the fair"
50. "Somewhere...over the rainbow"
51. "London bridge is...falling down"
52. "Oh, how I hate to get up...in the morning"
53. "There'll be blue birds over...the white cliffs of Dover"
54. "It's a long way...to Tipperary"
55. "Hail, hail...the gang's all here"
56. "For he's a jolly...good fellow"
57. "Happy birthday...to you"
58. "I'm dreaming of a ...white Christmas"
59. "In your Easter bonnet...with all the frills upon it"
60. "Or would you like to swing...on a star"
61. "Where the blue of the night...meets the gold of the day"
62. "Button up your...overcoat"
63. "I'm singing in the...rain"
64. "Oh, the weather outside is...frightful"
65. "I'm always chasing...rainbows"
66. "I'm forever blowing...bubbles"
67. "California...here I come"
68. "Nothin' could be finer than to be in...Carolina in the morning"
69. "Come away with me, Lucile, in my...merry Oldsmobile"
70. "See the U.S.A. in your...Chevrolet"
71. "She's only a bird in a...gilded cage"
72. "Every time it rains, it rains...pennies from heaven"
73. "This land is...your land"
74. "When it's springtime in the...Rockies"
75. "I'll be with you in...apple blossom time"
76. "Well, I went downtown for to see my gal, singing...polly wolly doodle all the day"
77. "By the light...of the silvery moon"
78. "Shine on, shine on...harvest moon"
79. "The leaves of brown came tumbling down, remember...in September in the rain"

80. "Wait 'til the sun shines...Nellie"
81. "Won't you come home...Bill Bailey"
82. "Though April showers may come your way, they bring the...flowers that bloom in May"
83. "Mary had a ...little lamb"
84. "You're a grand old flag...you're a high-flying flag"
85. "Oh, my name is McNamara...I'm the leader of the band"
86. "Give my regards to...Broadway"
87. "Have you ever seen a dream walking?...Well, I did"
88. "I'm a Yankee...doodle dandy"
89. "Oh, beautiful, for...spacious skies"
90. "Oh, say can you see...by the dawn's early light"
91. "My country...'tis of thee"
92. "Over the river and...through the woods"
93. "Yankee Doodle went to London...just to ride the ponies"
94. "God bless America...land that I love"
95. "Nights are long since...you went away"
96. "Glory, glory...hallelujah"
97. "Down in the...valley"
98. "Oh, I come from Alabama with my...banjo on my knee"
99. "Carolina moon...keep shining"
100. "I don't want to walk...without you, baby"

Name That Tune

The songs listed above can also be used for Name That Tune. This game can be played in a number of ways:

1. The leader hums the melody to the song or plays it on an instrument and the participants try to guess the song's name.

2. The leader sings all of the words except for the title and the participants guess the title.

3. The leader starts the song and the participants get credit for singing the rest of the words to the song, even if they cannot guess the title.

4. The leader hums the first part of the song and the participants hum the rest of it.

This game is very easily adapted to the abilities and needs of the participants. We've played this game in all of the ways described above at the AFCC, which made the game appropriate for persons who are quite impaired cognitively.

I don't usually begin by giving out the rules. I simply say, *"Let's play Name That Tune. I'll hum (or play) a melody and let's see if you recognize the song."* By using the word "recognize," I'm not asking for the song's name, so participants feel free to say, "Oh, I know that one!" or to hum the rest of the melody, even if they can't come up with the title. Participants don't feel they've failed, but that they've succeeded—after all, they do recognize the song.

I'll sometimes give hints: *"I can see you know the song's tune. The title is 'Let Me Call You...?'"* and nine times out of ten, someone in the group can finish the title. We'll often go on to sing (or hum) the whole song.

Parachute Dancing

The parachute is another favorite activity at the AFCC. It's bright and pretty and the breeze it provides is refreshing.

It's fun to choreograph movements with the parachute and to sing songs that serve as cues to the movements. We usually sit while using the parachute, as a few AFCC participants have poor balance. We also avoid right/left movements, since this can be confusing to the person with dementia. The participants who are sitting directly across from the leader tend to mirror what the leader does; so, if the leader is moving to the right, the participants across the circle will move to the left. This makes for some very disorganized choreography!

We use the following movements: lifting the parachute up over our heads, putting it down to the floor, rippling it (shaking it quickly up and down), pulling it towards ourselves, and pushing it away from ourselves. A typical choreography would look like this, with the top line representing the choreography:

"My Bonnie"

DOWN— UP— RIPPLE
My Bonnie lies over the ocean,

DOWN— UP— RIPPLE
My Bonnie lies over the sea.

DOWN— UP— RIPPLE
My Bonnie lies over the ocean,

DOWN— UP—
Oh bring back my Bonnie to me.

PULL— PUSH—
Bring back, bring back,

PULL— PUSH—
Oh bring back my Bonnie to me, to me.

PULL— PUSH—
Bring back, bring back,

PULL— PUSH.
Oh bring back my Bonnie to me.

"Daisy, Daisy"

UP— DOWN—PULL— PUSH—
Daisy, Daisy, give me your answer do.

UP— DOWN—PULL— PUSH—
I'm half crazy all for the love of you.

UP— DOWN—
It won't be a stylish marriage,

PULL— PUSH—
I can't afford a carriage.

UP— DOWN—
But you'll look sweet upon the seat

PULL— PUSH.
Of a bicycle built for two.

Follow the Bouncing Balloon

I don't know what it is about big, bright party balloons, but they're always a hit at the AFCC. There are many advantages to using balloons rather than inflatable or foam balls. First of all, balloons move more slowly, giving persons with coordination difficulties a bit more time to prepare to catch or hit them. A balloon's path through space is unpredictable. You may hit it hard in one direction, only to have it go in another direction or to move only a few feet. This quality seems to keep the group more focused—because who knows where the thing will end up? Balloons don't hurt and they rarely hit anyone with enough force to knock off glasses or dislodge hearing aids. This is reassuring to the visually impaired person who may not see the balloon until it's very close to him/her.

This is also important if there is a participant in the group who doesn't know his/her own strength: even if s/he hits the balloon with a great deal of force, it's unlikely to hurt anyone.

How to Play: This game requires a leader and a referee. The participants sit in two rows of chairs that face each other, with a piece of tape on the floor dividing the space in two.

You'll need a recording of active music. Some suggestions: Big Band music or one of the "Hooked on..." collections (I personally like "Hooked on Swing"). The music has to be loud enough to hear above the din of the game, but not so loud as to be overstimulating.

The leader starts the tape and the teams begin batting the ball back and forth. The leader should have his/her back to the game (that's why you need a referee) and should cut off the tape every 30 seconds or so. The team that has the balloon on their side of the tape then gets a point. The object of the game is to have the lowest score at the end, thereby encouraging the teams to KEEP THE BALLOON MOVING AT ALL TIMES away from their side of the line.

Music Trivia

Music trivia can be played in a number of ways. The leader can simply read the questions to the group one by one and have the group answer them. Another option is to write the categories on a board and allow individuals to pick their favorite category; they are then given a chance to answer the question, and if they can't, anyone in the group can. A third option is to number the categories 1-6 and have individuals roll a die. The number on the die will correspond to a category and the person will get a question from that category. Or, each person rolls the die, but anyone in the group can answer the question. Again, this group is adaptable to the many needs and abilities of the participants.

I usually begin the group by explaining that "trivia" means "unimportant" and that some of the questions are easy to answer, some hard. Mainly, we're here to have fun, not to test anyone's musical knowledge.

For some of the categories, you may need to give extra hints. For example, for the question, "What singer was fired by Arthur Godfrey on live TV?," many of the AFCC participants remembered the incident but not the singer's name. So, I said, "His first name was Julius," and several people shouted, "LaRosa!"

Category One: Complete the Line. For this category, pick 20 or so of the songs from the "Complete the Line" game listed earlier in this chapter.

Category Two: Bands/Singers

1. Who was known as "The Voice" in the 1940s? **Answer:** Frank Sinatra
2. Who was known as "Der Bingle"? **Answer:** Bing Crosby
3. What bandleader started his songs by saying, "A-one-ana-two"? **Answer:** Lawrence Welk
4. What instrument did Arthur Godfrey play? **Answer:** Ukelele
5. Whose theme song was "Take the 'A' Train"? **Answer:** Duke Ellington
6. What instrument did Duke Ellington play? **Answer:** Piano

7. What instrument did Benny Goodman play? **Answer:** Clarinet

8. What was the name of Guy Lombardo's orchestra? **Answer:** The Royal Canadians

9. What was Wayne King's nickname? **Answer:** The Waltz King

10. What bandleader was killed in a plane crash in WWII? **Answer:** Glenn Miller

11. Whose theme song was "Begin the Beguine"? **Answer:** Artie Shaw

12. Name a "sister group." **Answer:** Andrews, King, Lennon, or McGuire

13. What were the Andrews Sisters' first names? **Answer:** Patti, Maxene, and La Verne

14. What singer was fired by Arthur Godfrey on live TV? **Answer:** Julius LaRosa

15. Who sang "When the Moon Comes Over the Mountain"? **Answer:** Kate Smith

16. Who sang "The Tennessee Waltz"? **Answer:** Patti Page

17. What instrument did Glenn Miller play? **Answer:** Trombone

18. What instrument is sometimes called "the licorice stick"? **Answer:** Clarinet

19. Who was called "Lonesome George"? **Answer:** George Gobel

Category Three: Musical Instruments

For this category, show a picture of a musical instrument and have the person identify it. You can purchase musical instrument flash cards from many of the music companies listed in the resource list of this book.

Category Four: Signature Songs

"I'm going to tell you the name of a song. Please tell me what singer, star, or band is known for performing this song." Option: Play recordings, if you have them.

1. "Thanks For the Memories" – **Bob Hope**
2. "This Is My Song" – **Patti Page**
3. "Everybody Loves Somebody Sometime" – **Dean Martin**
4. "White Christmas" – **Bing Crosby**
5. "The Boogie Woogie Bugle Boy" – **Andrews Sisters**
6. "When the Moon Comes Over the Mountain" – **Kate Smith**
7. "Come On-a My House" – **Rosemary Clooney**
8. "I Left My Heart in San Francisco" – **Tony Bennett**
9. "(You Ain't Nothin' but a) Hound Dog" – **Elvis Presley**
10. "In the Mood" – **Glenn Miller**
11. "Stormy Weather" – **Lena Horne**
12. "Inka Dinka Doo" – **Jimmy Durante**
13. "Over the Rainbow" – **Judy Garland**
14. "Que Será, Será" – **Doris Day**
15. "A-Tisket, A-Tasket" – **Ella Fitzgerald**
16. "On the Good Ship Lollipop" – **Shirley Temple**
17. "Mister Bojangles" – **Sammy Davis, Jr.**
18. "My Kind of Town (Chicago is)" – **Frank Sinatra**
19. "Swanee" – **Al Jolson**
20. "Auld Lang Syne" – **Guy Lombardo and the Royal Canadians**

Category Five: Movies and Musicals

This is a tough category! You may want to give a few choices or cues for each question.

1. In what movie did Judy Garland sing "Over the Rainbow"? **Answer:** *The Wizard of Oz*
2. What was the name of the musical about the von Trapp family? **Answer:** *The Sound of Music*
3. What was the name of the movie in which Bing Crosby first sang "White Christmas"? Answer: *Holiday Inn*
4. In what musical did Mary Martin play a boy who could fly and never wanted to grow up? **Answer:** *Peter Pan*
5. Who was the sexy actress who starred with Crosby and Hope in the "Road" pictures? **Answer:** Dorothy Lamour
6. Who was the female movie star known for her talent in water ballet? **Answer:** Esther Williams
7. What musical introduced the songs "Some Enchanted Evening" and "Bali Ha'i"? **Answer:** *South Pacific*
8. What musical was based on the play *Anna and the King of Siam*? **Answer:** *The King and I*
9. What musical told the story of Tevye in the fictional Russian village Anatevka? **Answer:** *Fiddler on the Roof*
10. Who was Dean Martin's nutty partner? **Answer:** Jerry Lewis
11. What Judy Garland movie musical is about an unknown singer who becomes a star? **Answer:** *A Star is Born* or *Easter Parade*
12. What was the name of the first "talkie," which starred Al Jolson? **Answer:** *The Jazz Singer*
13. What male dancer starred in *Singing in the Rain* and *An American in Paris*? **Answer:** Gene Kelly
14. What musical is named after a state in the southwest? **Answer:** *Oklahoma*
15. Who is the 1930s child star who grew up to be a U.S. ambassador to Ghana? **Answer:** Shirley Temple
16. What U.S. president acted in *Knute Rockne, All-American* and *Bedtime for Bonzo*? **Answer:** Ronald Reagan
17. Who was Fred Astaire's most frequent dancing partner? **Answer:** Ginger Rogers
18. What female Latin singer and comedienne was known for her edible headgear? **Answer:** Carmen Miranda
19. What was the name of Roy Roger's horse? **Answer:** Trigger

Category Six: Potpourri

1. What bandleader hosted the show "The Kollege of Musical Knowledge"? **Answer:** Kay Kaiser
2. Name the Marx brothers. **Answer:** Harpo, Groucho, Chico, and Zeppo
3. Which Marx brother was an accomplished musician and took his nickname from the instrument he played? **Answer:** Harpo
4. Which sister group recorded "Bei Mir Bist Du Schön"? **Answer:** The Andrews Sisters

5. Which sister group recorded "Mairzy Doats"? **Answer**: The King Sisters

6. In "Put on Your Old Grey Bonnet," what's the horse's name? **Answer**: Dobbin

7. In "When You Wore a Tulip," what kind of a flower was the singer wearing? **Answer**: A big red rose

8. In the song "School Days," what was written on the slate? **Answer**: "I love you, Joe"

9. Name a woodwind instrument. **Answer**: Flute, clarinet, oboe, bassoon, saxophone, piccolo, or English horn

10. What instrument is on the singer's knee in "Oh! Susanna"? **Answer**: Banjo

11. How many keys are on a piano? **Answer**: 88

12. What are piano keys traditionally made of? **Answer**: Ebony and ivory

13. What's the smallest instrument in the orchestra, looking like a little flute? **Answer**: Piccolo

14. Name the four voices (parts) in a traditional choir. **Answer**: Soprano, alto, tenor, and bass

15. How many singers are in a quartet? **Answer**: Four

16. How many instruments are in an octet? **Answer**: Eight

17. What's the title of the person who leads a symphony orchestra? **Answer**: Conductor or maestro

19. Name a brass instrument. **Answer**: Trumpet, cornet, tuba, baritone, French horn, trombone

20. Name a keyboard instrument. **Answer**: Piano, harpsichord, organ, celeste

21. What's the name of the instrument you hum into to produce a buzzing noise? **Answer**: Kazoo

Chapter 10

Songwriting

General Goals

1. Opportunity for creative self-expression
2. Opportunity for choice
3. Increase self-esteem through participation in a structured, nonthreatening activity
4. Increase awareness of self, others

The Main Group at the AFCC has written many of its own songs. Earlier in the book, I mentioned the song we wrote called "I Feel Lousy." We've rarely written songs entirely from the top of our heads like that one, but we have employed the technique of lyric substitution to write songs.

Lyric Substitution

This simply means substituting your own words for the words of the song. This is what we've all done when we've sung song parodies, like this one for "Let Me Call You Sweetheart," which I learned from an older man I once worked with:

Don't you call me sweetheart!
I don't love you anymore,
Since I caught you necking
With the girl next door.
You think you're pretty special,
But you're just a bore!
Don't you call me sweetheart!
I don't love you anymore.

When using this technique, it doesn't work well to write the lyrics to the whole song on a board, leaving a few blanks here and there. This is pretty confusing for the person with dementia, who is likely to give you the original words to the song. Rather, treat the exercise like a word game. Ask the group for a type of word, like "a color" or "an adjective" or "a verb ending with -ing." Write these words down for yourself. You can later explain what you wanted the words for and can then "fill in the blanks" on a large board for the group to see.

For example, here's how we wrote a parody of "Yes, We Have No Bananas." I asked the group to tell me their favorite foods, preferably ethnic foods or foods with weird names. In the end, I told them we were collecting these words for a song and sang it to the group. I then wrote their word suggestions on a board for everyone to read. We came up with this:

Yes, we have no spaghetti,
We have no pizza today.
But we have lettuce, kohlrabi,
And celery and pickles,
And ice cream and apple pie;
We have an old-fashioned cube steak,
Long Island fruit cake,
But yes, we have no kumquats,
And no hasenpfeffer today.

You can do the same thing for the song, "My Favorite Things." Ask the group to name their favorite things. It works best if you have a list of categories to help focus people:

- Favorite color
- Favorite food
- Favorite girl's name
- Favorite boy's name
- Favorite holiday
- Favorite season
- Favorite vacation spot

Then, simply substitute this list for the original lyrics. You may need to take poetic license and add or subtract a word or two to make this work, but the end result may look like this (the words in parentheses are my additions):

(Big) yellow (flowers)
And hot dogs and French fries,
(Girl's name of) Ellen
And (boy's name of) Henry.
Christmas and summer and Miami Beach,
These are a few of my favorite things.

Silly Songs/Nonsensical Songs

To write a silly song, simply take a familiar song and delete words here and there. Begin the group by asking the participants to give you different kinds of words—the more unusual, the better. After the list is finished, fill in the words on a large piece of paper for everyone to read and sing the "silly song" you've just written. Here are a couple sample songs to use:

When You Wore a (?)

(Tune: "When You Wore a Tulip")

When you wore a (thing)
A big (color) (kitchen utensil)
And I wore a (size) (color) (clothing accessory)
When you (verb ending in -ed) me
'Twas then (place) (verb ending in -ed) me
What a (thing), no one knows.
You made life (adjective) when you called me (funny nickname)
'Twas down where the (color) (plant) grows,
Your (body part) was/were sweeter than (food)
When you wore a (thing you'd find in a bathroom)
And I wore a (size) (color) (thing)

Home on the (?)

(Tune: "Home on the Range")

Oh, give me a (place) where the (professional person) (action verb)
And the (professional sports team) and the (professional sports team) play,
Where seldom is heard a (funny noise) or a (funny noise)
And the (sports equipment) are not (adjective) all day.
Home, home on the (kitchen appliance),
Where the (insect) and the (insect) play,
Where seldom is heard a (adjective) word,
And the (food, plural) are not (adjective) all day.

Chapter 11

Sing-Alongs

General Goals

1. Opportunity for creative self-expression
2. Opportunity for socialization
3. Increase awareness of self, others
4. Increase self-esteem through participation in a structured, nonthreatening activity
5. Opportunity for choice

When I first began working at the AFCC, I tried to avoid sing-alongs because I felt they weren't therapeutic enough. With my head full of music therapy theory, I planned (what I thought were) creative, unique music groups. Unfortunately, these groups met my needs rather than the participants' needs. They most often just wanted to sing their favorite songs. Now every music group at the AFCC includes some time for group singing. The AFCC participants will put up with my ideas for music groups as long as I include group singing time as a part of them.

Singing feels good. It's a way to release tension, as Mrs. S points out:

"When I feel really tense, I go someplace by myself and sing my lungs out. Now, I can't carry a tune in a bucket, but it makes me feel like a million bucks."

♪

Singing is a very social activity. Singing usually occurs in social situations—in religious services, parties, as part of celebrations. There's something reassuring about group singing; it fosters a sense of belonging and community.

Persons with dementia have unique needs that need to be addressed in sing-alongs. First of all, persons with dementia may have a difficult time using songsheets properly. Some people may become distracted by them, shuffling through them, rolling them up, or folding them. Some people may not be able to read and may be embarrassed at being handed a songsheet they cannot use. You may notice individuals who pretend to read the words, but who are on the wrong page or who are holding the songsheet upside down. For these reasons, if you must use songsheets, I personally advocate using song lyric posters or overhead transparencies of song lyrics, both of which you can make yourself. In this way, individuals who are able to read can benefit from seeing the words to the songs, and you've removed a potential distracter for those persons who cannot use songsheets.

If you prefer to use individual songsheets over song lyric posters or slides, the following design tips may be helpful to you:

1. **One Song Per Page.** Print only one song per page. In this way, there will be no confusion about which song to sing.
2. **Use Upper- and Lowercase Letters.** It's easier for persons with visual impairments to read written materials printed in both upper- and lowercase letters than it is for them to read materials written in all uppercase (capital) letters. Uppercase letters can blur and begin to look alike to a person with a visual impairment. If you don't have access to a computer or a large-print typewriter, print the songs out by hand.
3. **Use One Page at a Time.** Hand out the songsheets as you use them. You can't hand out a ten-page songsheet and expect a group of persons with dementia to find the correct page and stick to it; it's simply too distracting. If you must use individual songsheets, hand out one page at a time and collect the last page before you hand out the new page. This way, everyone will have the right lyrics in front of them.
4. **Avoid Illustrations.** They're too distracting. It seems like a good idea to illustrate Christmas songsheets with pictures of Christmas trees or Santa Claus, but the illustrations can distract the person with dementia from the lyrics on the songsheet.
5. **Consider Not Using Songsheets at All.** I frequently avoid the use of songsheets altogether. AFCC sing-alongs focus on the participants' favorite songs, which they know quite well. I begin sing-alongs by emphasizing that it's not important that all of the words to the songs are sung; it's okay to just hum the tune. It's been my experience that persons who have difficulty remembering the words to familiar songs are not helped much by songsheets.

Sing-Along Ideas

1. **"Pass-the-hat" sing-along.** Persons with dementia are often unable to give requests for songs; it's difficult for them to spontaneously come up with a song title. For those who cannot name a song they'd like to hear, write song titles on small slips of paper and put them into a hat. Then, have a participant pull a slip out of the hat and read it to you or give it to you for you to read. Play the song chosen, then pass the hat to the next participant.
2. **Theme sing-alongs.** Plan a sing-along around a theme. Include some time for discussion. If you include props, you could plan an entire discussion/sensory stimulation session around these songs. (See Chapter 8, "Reminiscence Groups," page 42, for ideas.)

Flower/Plant Songs

"When You Wore a Tulip"
"Sweet Violets"
"My Wild Irish Rose"
"Jeannine, I Dream of Lilac Time"
"Daisy, Daisy"
"Tiptoe Through the Tulips"
"I'm a Lonely Little Petunia"
"Don't Sit Under the Apple Tree"

"I'm Looking Over a Four-Leaf Clover"
"Maple Leaf Rag"
"I'll Be With You in Apple Blossom Time"
"Second Hand Rose"

Women's Names

"Daisy, Daisy"
"K-K-K-Katy"
"I'll Take You Home Again, Kathleen"
"My Wild Irish Rose"
"Ida, Sweet as Apple Cider"
"Dinah"
"Sweet Adeline"
"Lil' Liza Jane"
"Mary's a Grand Old Name"
"Aura Lee"
"Cindy, Cindy"
"Wait 'Til the Sun Shines, Nellie"
"Alice Blue Gown"
"Once in Love with Amy"
"Toot, Toot, Tootsie"
"Minnie the Moocher"

Men's Names

"I'm Just Wild About Harry"
"Jimmy Crack Corn"
"When Johnny Comes Marching Home"
"Sonny Boy"
"Won't You Come Home, Bill Bailey"
"My Bill"
"Danny Boy"
"Alexander's Ragtime Band"
"Tom Dooley"
"My Buddy"
"Harrigan"
"Oh Johnny, Oh Johnny, Oh!"

Food and Drink

"Yes, We Have No Bananas"
"Don't Sit Under the Apple Tree"
"Beer Barrel Polka"
"Hot-Diggety-Dog"
"Rum and Coca-Cola"
"Animal Crackers in My Soup"
"Life is Just a Bowl of Cherries"
"Good Ship Lollipop"

Silly Songs

"The Flat Foot Floogie"
"Mairzy Doats"
"I Knew an Old Lady"
"Barney Google"
"Yes, We Have No Bananas"
"Hut Sut Song"
"Ma, He's Makin' Eyes at Me"
"Funny Face"
"Show Me the Way to Go Home"
"Ain't We Got Fun?"
"How Much is that Doggie in the Window?"
"Gimme a Little Kiss"

Colors

"The Yellow Rose of Texas"
"The White Cliffs of Dover"
"When the Red, Red Robin"
"Blue Skies"
"That Old Black Magic"
"Green, Green Grass of Home"
"Put on Your Old Grey Bonnet"
"The Old Grey Mare"
"Alice Blue Gown"
"Sweet Georgia Brown"
"Bye, Bye, Blackbird"
"My Blue Heaven"
"Green Eyes"
"Mood Indigo"
"Where the Blue of the Night"
"White Christmas"
"Red Sails in the Sunset"
"Blue Hawaii"
"By the Light of the Silvery Moon"
"Beautiful Brown Eyes"

Places

"Yellow Rose of Texas"
"Deep in the Heart of Texas"
"Bali Ha'i"
"Blue Hawaii"
"Oklahoma"
"Chicago (That Toddlin' Town)"
"April in Paris"
"Chattanooga Choo Choo"
"Over the Rainbow"
"Carolina Moon"
"42nd Street"
"Lullaby of Broadway"
"Over There"
"Beautiful Ohio"
"Swanee"
"Dixie"
"Georgia on My Mind"
"St. Louis Blues"
"How Are Things in Glocca Morra?"
"Sidewalks of New York"
"How Ya Gonna Keep 'Em Down on the Farm"
"I Left My Heart in San Francisco"

3. **"Balloon Buster" sing-along.** Write song titles on small pieces of paper and stuff the song titles into balloons before you inflate them. Each participant that desires can pop a balloon and retrieve the song title. The group then sings that song.

4. **"All Time Favorites" sing-along.** Select a group of songs for the group to sing. Have the participants vote on their top ten favorites. At a later session, tape the group singing their top ten favorites. In this way, you'll have a "Greatest Hits" tape available for the participants to enjoy hearing later.

Chapter 12

Music Groups for Lower-functioning Persons with Dementia

Working with "The Sensory Group"

AFCC participants are placed in the Sensory Group because of the following strengths and needs:

The Sensory Group: Strengths

1. Ability to interact with others one-to-one
2. Ability to interact with the environment in a meaningful way
3. Usually in excellent physical health
4. Aware of changes in the environment
5. Able to participate in ADLs with cuing, assistance

The Sensory Group: Needs

1. A calm, predictable environment
2. Sensory stimulation to prevent total withdrawal from the environment
3. One-to-one interaction in order to participate in recreational activities and activities of daily living
4. Assistance with communication
5. Assistance with physical coordination, possibly necessitating the use of cues, physical prompts, and/or adaptive devices/techniques
6. Activities designed to accommodate the symptoms of distractibility and shortened attention span

Although this description of the criteria of Sensory Group participants appears bleak, these individuals are capable of doing much more than we health care professionals often give them credit for. For example, Mr. J fits most of the above criteria. However, he's far from being a passive, useless human being. He has severe problems with word finding and his speech is often difficult to understand, but with a bit of time and patience from the listener, he's able to communicate. One of his favorite music activities is the "Complete the Line" group listed on pages 57-59. He isn't always able to sing the words perfectly but he knows the tunes, and the songs often start him reminiscing about past events that were important to him.

Mr. J also has a terrific sense of humor. As a warm-up, I'll sometimes read the first part of a proverb and ask Mr. J to finish it. One morning, after he'd correctly answered about a dozen proverbs, I began: "A bird in the hand...," to which he replied, laughing, "...is lousy!" Later, he finished "Behind every successful man" with "...is a nagging wife!"

Mrs. T also fits all of the Sensory Group criteria. She rarely speaks at all. During the activity mentioned above, she was sitting in a chair across from Mr. J and me and she appeared not to be paying attention. However, after we'd finished the phrase "Man does not live by bread alone," she asked, "Ya got any?" I took this as a cue that it was time to serve the morning snack.

It's been my experience that even persons in the later stages of dementing illnesses are able to comprehend at least some of what is going on around them. I've been surprised time and time again at the ability of extremely cognitively-impaired individuals to interpret the mood of the environment, even if they have difficulty understanding verbal communication.

Mrs. M is one such individual. She has an extremely short attention span which interferes with her ability to follow complex conversations. She is very sensitive to the environment, however. Earlier in this book, I mentioned the day that I was tired and grouchy and Mrs. M perfectly described how I felt (even though I thought I was covering up my feelings). She is constantly surprising us with her gift of perception:

During the lunch hour, Mrs. M was pacing in the hallway, in tears. A staff member walked up to her and asked what was wrong, to which Mrs. M replied, "They don't like me. I don't understand it. Nobody wants to talk to me. I've never done anything to them. Some people can be so mean." The staff member reassured Mrs. M that no one meant her any harm and then led her back to her lunch table. When he saw who Mrs. M was seated with, he suddenly realized why she was so upset. Mrs. M, who loves to talk (and can in fact border on the hyperverbal), was seated with a group of nonverbal individuals. Mrs. M had perceived their nonresponsiveness to her friendly chatter as "the silent treatment," and could not understand what she had done to deserve this.

♪

Although Mrs. M misinterpreted the intent of the people at her table, one can certainly understand why she felt the way that she did. (We now try to seat at least one other verbal person at the table with her.)

I mentioned earlier in this book that the AFCC discourages keeping the diagnosis from the person with dementia. We will respect a family's wishes as far as not bringing it up to the person, but if the person asks questions about their diagnosis, we will answer them as honestly as possible. We firmly believe that the people with dementia are aware that something is wrong, even if they aren't told the diagnosis. We haven't decided this on our own; the participants have let us know this:

Mr. G noticed the word "Alzheimer's" on written materials his wife had at home. He asked, "Is this what I have?" His wife, who had avoided discussing this with him, said, "Yes, it is." Mr. G breathed a sigh of relief and said, "Thank God. I thought I was going crazy."

Mrs. M will occasionally hold her head and moan, "I don't know what's wrong. Sometimes I feel as if I'm losing my mind."

Mrs. T says, "Sometimes I just sit there [when there's a conversation going on] and I hope no one will ask me [a question] because I can't follow it."

Mrs. S says, "I was a living bitch until I found out what I've got. I knew something was wrong, but I didn't know what. Then when I found out, I stayed in bed for a year; I just couldn't face what was happening to me."

♪

The moral of the story: don't assume that people can't understand what is happening to them or that they can't understand what is going on around them. A person does not stop being a person once s/he is diagnosed with a dementing illness—not even in the later stages of the illness.

The Do's and Don't's of Working with Persons with Dementia

The following list, adapted from the work of Susan Quattrochi-Tubin, Ph.D., may be helpful to you when working with a person with advanced dementia:

Do:

1. **Treat the person as an adult.** Although the person with dementia is confused, s/he is an adult and deserves to be treated like one.
2. **Be sensitive to the environment.** Is it calm? Quiet? Is the temperature comfortable? Is the lighting too bright? An uncomfortable environment may be the cause of catastrophic reactions.
3. **Help the person to remain as independent as possible.** It may be quicker to do things for him/her, but it is better for the person to do things for himself/herself.
4. **Simplify instructions.** Give one direction at a time to avoid confusion.
5. **Establish a fixed routine.** A familiar schedule is very helpful.
6. **Speak to the person as if s/he understands.** Give the individual the benefit of the doubt. S/he may surprise you.
7. **Respond to the person's feelings,** not just the words expressed.
8. **Be flexible.** Creativity helps when working with the person with dementia.
9. **Learn as much about the person's past as you can.** This will help you immensely in planning programs and when calming a person who is upset.
10. **Give encouragement.** Imagine not knowing who you are or where you are. You'd need encouragement, too.
11. **Be patient.** Give the person extra time to respond to questions or requests. Do not bombard the person with multiple questions or requests. Rushing the person usually winds up frustrating both of you.

Don't:

1. **Speak to the person as if s/he were a child.** This can cause angry reactions and it indicates a lack of respect.

2. **Scold the person.** S/he is not intentionally making a mistake. Instead, quietly and gently point out the behavior and suggest an alternative.

3. **Speak to the person in negatives.** You'll get a better response if you say, "Come with me" than you will with, "You can't go there." Avoid negative phrases like, "Don't do that" or "You're doing it the wrong way."

4. **Startle the person.** Approach the person from the front. Be sure s/he sees you before you begin to speak.

5. **Assume that every person with dementia is the same.** Dementia progresses differently in different people.

6. **Be afraid to touch the person or give a hug once in a while.** Express some affection. The person with dementia likely does not get enough of it.

7. **Talk "around" a person with dementia, as if s/he isn't there.** S/he may understand more than you think.

8. **Give up!**

General Goals for Lower-functioning Clients

1. Opportunity for creative self-expression
2. Sensory stimulation
3. Increase awareness of self, others
4. Increase self-esteem through participation in a structured, nonthreatening activity
5. Opportunity for autonomy and decision making
6. Assess and maintain eye-hand coordination, fine- and gross-motor coordination, ability to read, ability to follow complex directions
7. Provide a means of nonverbal communication
8. Elicit extramusical associations (memories)

Adapting Higher-functioning Groups

It's difficult to run a "group" for persons who are in the later stages of a dementing illness. These persons often require one-to-one interaction in order to successfully participate in recreational activities or activities of daily living. At the AFCC, we often gather the individuals in the Sensory Group in a circle or around a table and go from person to person, repeating the activity or asking a question of each person. (There are no more than seven or eight persons in this group.)

When working with persons in the later stages of a dementing illness, you may need to scale down your expectations in terms of active participation in sessions. Perhaps a person never speaks, but sings a few words to a song, or sits with his/her eyes closed but opens them when music is played. These small attempts to interact with the environment are significant. Don't be discouraged if the person doesn't sing every word or doesn't reach out to play an instrument during a sensory stimulation session. For some individuals, simply watching the others in the room may be a significant interaction.

Persons in the later stages of a dementing illness may be easily overstimulated. When adapting music groups for these individuals, avoid stimulating more than two senses at a time. Try to keep the environment calm and reasonably quiet. Avoid groups that involve quick physical responses because these persons may have coordination problems that prevent them from responding quickly. Give only one instruction at a time and make sure the person understands the instruction before you continue.

Music Groups

Many of the groups in the previous section are appropriate for lower-functioning individuals, with minor adaptations:

Complete the Line

Persons who are in the later stages of dementing illnesses may not be able to sing the next line of the song, but may be able to sing, hum, or whistle the rest of the tune. Consider the activity a success if the person can hum the rest of the line, and extremely successful if the person can remember a few of the words (or the gist of the words, like answering "I love you" in response to "Let me call you sweetheart").

Name That Tune

Sing the tune, leaving out the title words. Give additional cues to encourage the person to remember the words. For example, for "My Blue Heaven," you may point to yourself, to something that is blue, and up towards the sky. Or you may give additional verbal cues: *"This song is 'My Blue...'?"*

Follow the Bouncing Balloon

You may need to simplify this game by simply bouncing the balloon around the group while instrumental music is playing. In my experience, instrumental music is best for background music; vocal music tends to distract the group from the leader's verbal instructions.

You'll definitely want to use a balloon rather than a foam ball or a beach ball. The bigger and slower the balloon, the better. Use a balloon that contrasts with the colors in the room so that it's easily seen. Give lots of physical cues: *"Look up, George...it's heading for you."*

Parachute Dancing

Use instrumental music as a background and encourage the group to move the parachute in sequence: up/down, side-to-side, or in/out. Concentrate on slow movements. Do one set of movements through the entire song, rather than switching movements mid-song. You will likely need a co-leader to successfully facilitate this group, as some individuals may need physical assistance to participate successfully in the session.

Sing-Alongs

Don't use songsheets. Don't concern yourself with the participants' ability to remember the words. Consider the sing-along a success if (1) the participants focus on your singing and perhaps sing along a bit with you, and (2) the participants hum along the tune, tap their feet in rhythm to the music, or in some nonverbal way indicate their attendance to the activity. After all, listening is a form of participation when it comes to music groups.

Chapter 13

Sensory Stimulation Groups

Sensory stimulation groups are designed to provide the withdrawn, passive individual with opportunities for interaction within a nonthreatening, supportive environment. The primary goal is to stimulate one or more senses within the session. The following groups focus mostly on visual, aural, and tactile stimulation, but olfactory and gustatory stimulation can be provided by offering a snack at the end of the session, if you choose to do so.

The goals in sensory stimulation groups are geared towards the individual participants. For example, Mr. S may be able to identify objects verbally; so a goal for him may be to correctly identify one object verbally. Mrs. N may not be able to verbally identify an object, but may be able to point to an object; so a goal for her may be to choose the correct object from a group of objects. Mr. P may not be able to do even this, so the goal for him may be to focus visually on the activity for ten minutes of the session.

Sensory stimulation groups should be done while sitting in a circle or around a table. In this way, the group leader can watch all of the participants, and the participants can watch one another.

Keep all of the materials that you will need for the group close to you so that you don't need to get up from your chair during the session. Persons in the later stages of a dementing illness tend to be very distractible, so you'll want to keep unnecessary movement down to a minimum.

Because of shortened attention spans, your group may not be able to tolerate an activity of longer than 20-30 minutes. If the participants become restless, move on to something else. The following groups are designed so that each individual step can be used as an independent, short activity, if needed.

Colors

Materials Needed

Sheets of construction paper in the following colors: red, white, blue, yellow, green, black, brown, light blue, pink, orange, and purple. If you can find them, use cellophane sheets of the three primary colors: red, yellow, and blue (check teachers' stores and art supply stores). If you play an accompanying instrument, keep it nearby.

Procedure

Introduction. Introduce the topic of colors. Begin by asking the participants to name a few colors. It may be helpful to point out things in the room and ask the participants to name the color of the object(s).

Color identification. Show the participants the pieces of construction paper, one at a time, and ask them to identify the colors. Ask if there is anything that they can think of that comes in that color, e.g., yellow bananas, red apples, etc.

Color combinations. Show the participants the following colors and ask them if they can think of anything that comes in these color combinations:

- Red, white, and blue: the American, British flags
- Red, yellow, and green: a stoplight
- Red and white: a stop sign, a barber pole, a candy cane
- Black and white: a newspaper, piano keys, skunks, zebras
- Light blue and pink: baby colors (blue for boys; pink for girls), spring and Easter colors

Color mixes. Show the participants the cellophane sheets of the primary colors (red, yellow, and blue). Discuss how all colors are a mixture of these three basic colors. Then, taking two of the colors, ask what color they think will be the result when they're mixed. After the participants have given their answers, layer the cellophane sheets and hold them up to the light so that the participants can see the result.

- Red and blue = purple
- Blue and yellow = green
- Red, yellow, and blue = brown
- Red and yellow = orange

Music. Play songs that have colors in them. Ask the participants to sing the songs, if they'd like to, and to identify the color that was sung. Choose short songs, where the color is obvious, or sing the first verse only. Suggested songs:

"When the Red, Red Robin Comes Bob-Bob-Bobbin' Along"
"Yellow Rose of Texas"
"Little Brown Jug"
"The Old Grey Mare"
"Baa, Baa Black Sheep"

"My Blue Heaven"
"White Christmas"
"The Green, Green Grass of Home"
"Deep Purple"

You may want to show the participants a color chart and have them point out the color they heard in the song after they've verbally identified it.

Closure. Thank each individual for participating in the group. Close with a song that is familiar to the group and suggests closure, like "'Til We Meet Again," or you may choose to take liberties with song lyrics and sing one of these closing songs (or one of your own choice):

"Goodbye, My Friends"

(Tune: "Goodnight, Ladies")

Goodbye, my friends,
All things must end,
Goodbye, my friends,
I really hate to go.

"My Friends, Goodbye"

(Tune: "Irene, Goodnight")

Goodbye, my friends,
My friends, goodbye.
Goodbye, my friends, goodbye, my friends,
Our music group must end.

Flowers/Plants

Materials Needed

Silk or plastic replicas of the following flowers or plants (or real ones, if possible): roses, daisies, four-leaf clovers, lilacs, tulips, morning glories, violets, daffodils.

If you can't get replicas of these plants, find photos of them. (Look in gardening books or catalogs.) Additional props: small gardening tools such as trowels and weed-pullers, watering cans, gardening gloves, knee pads, seed packets, small pots (for indoor gardens), and potting soil.

Procedure

Introduction. Introduce the topic of flowers. Begin by asking the participants to name as many flowers as they can. It may help to ask questions:

1. What plants are associated with Christmas? **Answer:** poinsettias, mistletoe, holly, pine
2. Name some bulb plants that come up in the early spring. **Answer:** crocuses, tulips, daffodils, hyacinths, lilies-of-the-valley
3. If you really love someone, you may send him or her a dozen long-stemmed red what? **Answer:** roses
4. This plant is closely associated with Easter. **Answer:** Easter lily
5. Name a plant that smells good. **Answer:** roses, lilacs, lavender, geraniums, hyacinths, lilies-of-the-valley (and almost any plant, as pleasurable scents vary from person to person)
6. This four-leafed plant is supposed to bring you good luck. **Answer:** clover
7. This plant is associated with St. Patrick's Day. **Answer:** shamrock

Identification of flowers/plants. Show the flowers to the participants and ask them to identify each flower. Give cues, if necessary.

Props/tactile stimulation. Pass around the gardening items, one at a time. You may want to ask: *"Did you ever keep a garden? What did you grow in it? If you grew vegetables or fruits, did you do any canning? What tools did you use when tending to your garden? Did you enjoy gardening?"*

Music. Play songs that mention flowers or plants and ask the participants to sing the songs, if they'd like to, and to identify the flower or plant mentioned. Suggested songs:

"Yellow Rose of Texas"
"When You Wore a Tulip"
"Jeannine, I Dream of Lilac Time"
"Sweet Violets"
"I'm Looking over a Four-Leaf Clover"
"Daisy, Daisy"

You may want to show the participants the replicas or photos of flowers after each song, and ask them to match the flower(s) with the one(s) mentioned in the song.

Closure. Thank each individual for participating in the group. Sing a closing song.

The Seasons

Materials Needed

Photos of seasonal scenes, such as beach scenes for the summer, spring flowers for the spring, harvest scenes and changing colors for the fall, and snow scenes for the winter.

Props

- suntan lotion
- seed packets
- sunglasses
- gardening tools
- real or paper fall leaves
- school supplies
- scarves, hats, or gloves
- old greeting cards

Note: There's enough material in each of these sections for an entire group. You may want to focus on just one season per group session so as not to overwhelm the participants (or yourself). You also may want to use the appropriate session at the beginning of each season.

Procedure

Introduction. Introduce the topic of the seasons. Ask the group to identify the four seasons of the year.

"Summer" discussion. Show the photos of summer scenes to the participants and have them identify the season and the activity depicted in the photo(s). Discuss the photos: *"What is going on in this photo? Have you ever done this? Did you like doing this?*

Follow the photos with the appropriate props. Allow the participants to handle the props. If you're passing around a pair of sunglasses, let the participants try them on. If you're passing around a bottle of suntan lotion, pour a bit on the participants' hands and let them touch it or smell it.

Sing "In the Good Old Summertime." Encourage the participants to sing along. Discuss the song afterwards: *"What do you like to do in the summer? What do you do to cool off on a hot summer day?"*

Discuss holidays that occur in the summer: Independence Day and Labor Day. Show the greeting cards for the appropriate holidays to the group to help stimulate discussion.

Summer Holiday Quiz

1. When is Independence Day? **Answer:** July 4th
2. What do we celebrate on Independence Day? **Answer:** Signing of the Declaration of Independence
3. When is Labor Day? **Answer:** first Monday in September
4. What do you do to celebrate Labor Day? **Answer:** Take the day off; have a picnic or barbecue

Sing songs that are associated with these holidays such as "God Bless America" or "The Star Spangled Banner" for Independence Day and "I've Been Working on the Railroad" for Labor Day.

"Autumn" discussion. Show the photos of autumn scenes to the participants and have them identify the season and the activity depicted in the photos. Discuss the photos and what is going on in them.

Follow the photos with the autumn props. Discuss the props as you pass them around for the participants to handle. Sing the song "School Days" and discuss school. (For some ideas, see the "School Days" group description on pages 48-49.)

Discuss holidays that occur in autumn:

- Rosh Hashana
- Yom Kippur
- Veteran's Day
- Sukkoth
- Thanksgiving
- Election Day
- Columbus Day
- Halloween

Show the greeting cards for the appropriate holidays to the group to help stimulate discussion.

The Jewish High Holy Days occur in late September or October. Check your calendar for the exact dates in a given year. Jewish holidays begin at sundown; when non-Jewish calendars say "first day of..." the holiday usually begins the evening before. *Sukkoth* is a festival of thanks that commemorates the sheltering of the Jews in tents after the exodus from Egypt. *Rosh Hashana* is the Jewish New Year. *Yom Kippur*, or the Day of Atonement, is the most solemn day of the Jewish year. It's celebrated eight days after Rosh Hashana and is observed with fasting and prayers of repentance.

Autumn Holiday Quiz

1. When is Columbus Day? **Answer:** October 12
2. When is Halloween? **Answer:** October 31
3. What do we do to celebrate Halloween? **Answer:** dress in costumes, go trick-or-treating
4. When is Election Day? **Answer:** first Tuesday after the first Monday in November
5. When is Veterans Day? **Answer:** November 11
6. When is Thanksgiving? **Answer:** fourth Thursday in November
7. What kinds of food do you usually eat on Thanksgiving? **Answer:** Turkey, dressing, mashed potatoes, etc.

Sing songs associated with these holidays to elicit memories. For Veterans Day, you may want to sing the armed forces songs: "And the Caissons go Rolling Along" (army), "Anchors Aweigh" (navy), "Up We Go into the Wild Blue Yonder" (air force), "The Marine Hymn" (marines). For Thanksgiving, you could sing "Come, Ye Thankful People Come."

"Winter" discussion. As described in the "summer" and "autumn" discussions, show the photos and props to the participants and discuss them.

Sing the song "Let it Snow" and discuss things that you can do with the snow (snowball fights, building snowmen, making snow angels, shoveling snow, building snow forts, skiing, sledding, etc.). Note: If this session takes place on a snowy day, use real snow.

Discuss holidays that occur in the winter:

- Hanukkah
- Christmas
- New Year's Eve/Day
- Valentine's Day
- Washington's Birthday
- Lincoln's Birthday
- Martin Luther King, Jr. Day
- St. Joseph's Day
- St. Patrick's Day
- Ash Wednesday

Show the greeting cards for the appropriate holidays to the participants to help stimulate discussion.

Hanukkah, the Festival of Lights, commemorates the victory of the Jews over the Syrians in the second century B.C. (check your calendar for the exact date in a given year).

Winter Holiday Quiz

1. How many days and nights is Hanukkah celebrated? **Answer:** Eight
2. When is Christmas? **Answer:** December 25
3. When is New Year's Eve? **Answer:** December 31
4. What February holiday is associated with hearts and flowers? **Answer:** Valentine's Day, February 14
5. When is Lincoln's birthday? **Answer:** February 12
6. When is Washington's birthday? **Answer:** February 22
7. What March holiday is held in honor of the patron saint of Ireland? **Answer:** St. Patrick's Day (March 17)
8. What March holiday is held in honor of the patron saint of Italy and Poland? **Answer:** St. Joseph's Day (March 19th)
9. What January holiday is held in honor of a great civil rights leader? **Answer:** Martin Luther King, Jr., Day, the third Monday in January

Sing songs that are associated with winter holidays such as "My Dreydel" for Hanukkah, "Silent Night" for Christmas, "Auld Lang Syne" for New Year's Eve, "I Love You Truly" for Valentine's Day, "When Irish Eyes Are Smiling" for St. Patrick's Day.

"Spring" discussion. As described in the above three seasonal discussions, show the photos and props to the participants and discuss them.

Sing "When the Red, Red, Robin Comes Bob-Bob-Bobbin' Along." Discuss the different signs of spring: robins; tulips, crocuses, and other spring flowers; trees budding; warm weather.

Discuss holidays that occur in the spring using the greeting cards to help stimulate discussion:

- Palm Sunday
- Easter
- Passover
- Mother's Day
- Father's Day
- Memorial Day
- Flag Day

Passover is a Jewish festival commemorating the liberation of the Jews from slavery in Egypt.

Spring Holiday Quiz

1. For what holiday do we give baskets and look for eggs? **Answer**: Easter
2. When is April Fool's Day? **Answer**: April 1
3. What holiday is just for moms? **Answer**: Mother's Day (third Sunday in May)
4. What spring holiday honors the men and women who have died in American wars? **Answer**: Memorial Day (celebrated the last Monday in May)
5. What holiday celebrates the stars and stripes? **Answer**: Flag Day (June 14)
6. What holiday is just for dads? Answer: Father's Day (third Sunday in June)

Sing songs that are associated with these holidays such as silly songs for April Fool's Day, "M-O-T-H-E-R" for Mother's Day, "Easter Parade" for Easter.

Closure. Thank everyone for participating. Sing a closing song.

Using Percussion Instruments for Sensory Stimulation

Goals

1. Assess and maintain eye-hand coordination, fine- and gross-motor coordination
2. Provide a means of creative self-expression
3. Provide a means of nonverbal communication
4. Increase self-esteem through participation in positive experience

Earlier in this section of the book, I mentioned a research study conducted by Alicia Clair and Barry Bernstein that concluded that persons in the later stages of a dementing illness respond best to vibrotactile stimulation, which is tactile stimulation that includes the perception of vibration. Percussion (or rhythm) instruments are an excellent choice in terms of vibrotactile stimulation. Avoid instruments that are very loud, as they may startle lower-functioning individuals and possibly cause catastrophic reactions. Focus instead on instruments that are quieter or that produce pleasant sounds.

While not all-inclusive, the following list of rhythm instruments will give you some ideas as to what to use:

Hand drums are tambourines without cymbals. They sometimes come with handles to make them easier to hold.

Maracas, or shakers, are a Latin instrument that sounds like a rattle. Authentic maracas are made of dried gourds and are colorfully painted, which adds to their value as a sensory stimulation tool.

Jingle bells come in a variety of forms, from a few bells attached to a handle, to a multitude of bells sewn onto a wooden base. The larger jingle bells can get very noisy, so instead use the smaller, quieter ones.

Jingle taps consist of a stick with a pair of tiny cymbals (like the ones on a tambourine) attached to one end. Tapping the stick sounds the cymbals.

Claves are a pair of polished wooden sticks usually made of a good hardwood. When hit together, they produce a light, hollow clicking sound.

Lummi sticks are long claves usually made of an inexpensive wood. Usually one stick in the set is smooth while the other is grooved. You can hit them together to produce a clicking sound or rub them together to produce a grating sound.

Triangles are tuned, triangular pieces of metal. The triangle is suspended from a handle and hit with a mallet to produce a pleasant, bell-like sound.

Wood blocks, tick-tock blocks, temple blocks, and log drums are tuned percussion instruments that are played with a mallet. When struck they produce a sound that resembles a clock ticking or a galloping horse.

It would take an entire book to list every rhythm instrument that can provide vibrotactile stimulation. The above instruments are relatively inexpensive and easy to find. (For information on where to obtain these instruments, see the Appendix.)

Persons in the later stages of a dementing illness have poor impulse control and short attention spans. Remember this when using rhythm instruments for sensory stimulation. If you give every individual an instrument at the same time, you can expect that everyone will play their instruments at the same time, and that everyone (including you) will end up overstimulated and anxious from all of the noise and confusion.

Instead, look at the group as a series of one-to-one sessions. Take an instrument to one person in the group. Demonstrate the instrument to that person, then give it to him/her to play. After a few minutes, move on to the next person. By doing this, you've given each individual an opportunity for sensory stimulation and you've also demonstrated the use of the instrument so that group members who are watching the session may be able to perform the task from observations of others.

It's a good idea to observe not only the person with whom you are working, but also the others in the group. Clair and Bernstein suggest that cognitively-impaired people benefit from the observation of others' participation, particularly if they are not able to participate fully on their own.

To get the maximum benefit of vibrotactile stimulation, the person with whom you are working should hold the instrument while playing it, rather than playing it while it rests on a table. The following sensory stimulation exercises can provide vibrotactile stimulation and are listed in order of complexity:

1. **Music Lesson**. Demonstrate an instrument and then have the participant play it. Offer assistance if needed.

2. **Repeat after Me**. Play a rhythm on the instrument and then have the participant repeat it. Keep the rhythm simple. For example, hit the instrument twice; if the person can do this, then hit it in a steady beat while singing a song.

3. **Rhythm Band**. Demonstrate more complex rhythms and have the participant repeat them. For example, demonstrate a quarter-note, two eighth-notes rhythm: one, two-and/one, two-and. (Note: A quarter note is equal to one pulse to the beat; an eighth note equals two pulses to the beat.)

4. **Sounds Like**. Give a choice between two instruments. Which one sounds like (answers are in italics):

   - A gunshot (*a mallet on a hand drum* or a bell)

- A clock (*a tick-tock block or wood block* or a triangle)
- An alarm clock (*a jingle bell* or a hand drum)
- A horse (*claves or tick-tock blocks* or jingle bells)
- A sleigh (a triangle or *a jingle bell*)
- A dinner bell (claves or *a triangle*)

You may want to try several instruments throughout the session to see which persons respond the best to which instruments. One person who doesn't respond to the hand drum may respond to the triangle.

Using Other Instruments for Sensory Stimulation

Guitar: You can use the guitar as a vibrotactile stimulation tool by positioning the guitar across the lap of the person with whom you're working. Stand behind the person and assist him/her to strum the strings while you play the chords. If the person cannot strum the strings, you can; what is important is that the person feel the vibrations through the back of the guitar.

Autoharp: If you have access to an autoharp, position it in the lap of the person you are working with. Sit across from the person and strum the autoharp, perhaps while singing a song.

Omnichord: The Omnichord is an electronic version of the autoharp, made by the Suzuki musical instrument company. It plays rhythm patterns in addition to playing chords and has an adjustable volume. It's easy to play and I've used it with much success with this population. To use it for sensory stimulation, position it in the lap of the person you are working with. Sit across from the person and strum it, perhaps while singing a song. Experiment with the different features to see what the person responds to. Encourage the person to play the instrument.

Piano or electronic keyboard: Seat the person with whom you are working in front of the keyboard. Encourage him/her to touch the keys, perhaps to play a melody or chords (if the person has experience playing the piano). If the person feels comfortable playing, you may want to improvise an accompaniment or play chords to his/her melody.

Xylophone or tone bells: Set the instrument in front of the person and demonstrate how to play it. After you've demonstrated it, hand the mallet to the person and let him/her try it. Once the person has mastered hitting the instrument, play a simple pattern and ask the person to repeat it. It takes a great deal of coordination to play these instruments, and some late-stage persons may not be able to play them at all.

Occasionally, even the best-planned sensory stimulation session may be overstimulating to someone in your group. If you notice a group member becoming upset, more confused, or restless, discontinue the activity. You can always try it again another time.

Chapter 14

"The Walking Club": Working with Persons Who Need to Pace

AFCC participants are placed in the Walking Club because of one primary need—the need to pace.

It's been our experience at the AFCC that persons who pace seem to do best in an environment with other persons who pace. This constant motion can be distracting and upsetting to lower-functioning persons with dementia (like the AFCC's Sensory Group) and can be annoying to higher-functioning persons with dementia. People who pace, apparently, are not bothered by other people's pacing. That is why we have a separate, special program for these individuals.

Pacing is often mentioned in the dementia literature as a "problem behavior." In actuality, pacing is a symptom, not a behavior. We would never become impatient with a person who has the flu for running a fever or sneezing; we expect these things to happen because it's a part of the sickness. Likewise, we should expect that persons with dementia may develop the need to pace. If you've ever worked or lived with a person who paces, you know that the person is fine as long as s/he is moving. Difficulties arise when we try to restrict the person's movement or make him/her sit still.

Walking Club Participants: Strengths

1. Physically active
2. Aware of changes in the physical environment
3. Aware of other people in the environment
4. Spontaneously interactive with staff and one another
5. Able to seek out sensory-stimulating experiences

Walking Club Participants: Needs

1. Freedom to pace
2. Assistance in Activities of Daily Living
3. Adaptive techniques to promote independence
4. A calm environment to minimize potential for catastrophic reactions and to minimize distracters
5. Human contact
6. Sensory stimulation

7. Activities designed to accommodate the symptoms of distractibility and shortened attention span
8. Activities that can be done on the run

Most catastrophic reactions that occur in people who pace are a result of one of two things: (1) The person's need to pace is being restricted, or (2) the person is being made to do something s/he does not want to. When you work with persons who pace, take their lead. Trying to force them to sit or to do what you want them to do will only result in frustration on both sides.

Programming in the Walking Club accommodates the participants' need to pace. All programming is done on our feet. If a participant walks away, we'll gently redirect him/her to the activity. If s/he doesn't seem interested in the activity, we don't insist that s/he participate.

The walls in the Walking Club room are paneled with pegboard which is hung with a variety of objects: scarves, hats, jewelry, bags, towels, purses, pictures, etc. There are brochure and magazine racks along one side of the room that are filled with magazines, brochures, pamphlets, and papers. There is an upright piano along one wall and a series of benches along another. A long table with six chairs around it sits in the center of the room and a round table sits towards one corner. Along the other walls are comfortable armchairs. There is a carpet sweeper in one corner and a stereo in another. Except for the table, the center of the room is unobstructed, allowing lots of room to pace.

Because the room is full of interesting "stuff," including balloons, beach balls, and active game equipment, people who are not interested in an activity can always find something to examine, work with, or admire.

Music in the Walking Club

Music is an excellent activity for persons who wander or pace because music activities can be done on your feet. I will rarely be able to keep the "music group" close to me in the Walking Club, but people walk up to me, listen for a while, and then walk away. I can tell if a person is listening by observing him/her. Some people close their eyes and sway in time with the music. Some pace in rhythm to the music. Some hum the tunes to the songs. Nearly everyone claps their hands after a song is finished.

The activities listed for the Sensory Group can all be done in the Walking Club. The only difference is that you will need to be on your feet, bringing the materials from person to person, since there is only a slight chance that the participants will be able to sit together for more than a few minutes at a time.

People who pace may develop "hoarding" behaviors. These individuals like to collect things; their pockets may be stuffed with napkins and slips of paper, and they may walk about with their arms full of things. This is a relatively benign behavior, but can be a problem if (1) you have items in the activity area that could potentially be dangerous, and (2) you have items in the activity area that you do not want the person to walk off with.

If a person who hoards latches onto an item you'd like back, you may be able to get it back by simply asking for it (*"I see you're holding my purse, Mrs. D. May I have it back?"* or *"You found my book, Mr. S. Thank you!"*). If the person continues to hold onto the item, try trading it for another item. If this doesn't work, just wait. The person will eventually put everything down and start hoarding again. Your best bet is to never leave out items that you can't afford to lose.

Using Rhythm Instruments

Playing rhythm instruments is an excellent activity because it works with the participants' need to move. Try the activities listed under "Sensory Stimulation" in the previous section. You'll probably need to work with each individual one at a time and will likely be doing the activities while walking.

After you've demonstrated the use of an instrument and after the person has learned how to play it, you may want to play the same instrument along with the person while singing a song together. For example, you may both be playing the jingle bells while singing "Jingle Bells," or may both play the hand drum while singing "When Johnny Comes Marching Home."

Dancing

People who pace may enjoy dancing. Don't worry if the person's sense of rhythm is off or if s/he doesn't remember the steps. The person may just move back and forth while you swing his/her arms.

Mr. K loved to dance. When two musicians came to entertain at a party, Mr. K jumped out of his seat and began swaying back and forth, smiling. A staff member led him to the aisle and "danced" with him. Although he couldn't communicate verbally, his body language indicated that he enjoyed the dancing very much.

A staff member took Mrs. S's hands and moved her arms back and forth to a slow waltz number. When the song was finished, Mrs. S, who did not seem to be particularly aware that music was playing, looked at the staff member and said, "Thanks, that was lovely."

♪

Try playing slow waltz tunes and swaying the person's arms from side to side. If the person with whom you're working remembers how to dance, let him/her lead. You may also want to try playing polkas or two-step tunes, since these are relatively simple dances.

Overstimulation

Loud music can be overstimulating for people who pace. These individuals are easily distracted and may have an extremely short attention span. Be careful that the music isn't too loud and the movement isn't too fast. If you notice anyone becoming anxious or upset, stop the activity.

I was playing "Down By the Riverside" on the piano for Mrs. L, who was smiling and singing along. When the song was finished, Mrs. S walked up to the piano. As I prepared to play another song, Mrs. S said, "That's enough of that!"

♪

Mrs. S. was pretty clear about her feelings. The music was too much for her at that moment, so I stopped playing until later, when I began with a quieter song.

Encouraging Participants to Use Musical Instruments for Self-Stimulation

The Walking Club participants use materials in the room for self-stimulation when the activity that is going on does not hold their attention. Consider using musical instruments with persons who pace, but be careful about the quality and type of instrument you make available to them.

First of all, make sure that the instruments provided for self-stimulation will not be dangerous if broken. Persons who pace have a tendency to take things apart and to drop things. You'll want to make sure that if the instruments break, there will be no sharp edges or points that could cause an injury.

Make sure the instruments are not terribly loud. You may notice that I did not mention the tambourine in the section on rhythm instruments and sensory stimulation. This is because the tambourine is a loud instrument, which may startle the person with dementia and cause a catastrophic reaction. Concentrate instead on bells, small drums, tick-tock or wood blocks, triangles, and lummi sticks.

You may want to purchase a small xylophone and mount it on the wall with a mallet suspended from a string nearby. Xylophones are relatively inexpensive, quiet, and pleasant-sounding.

You may also want to purchase a set of tubular wind chimes. Tubular chimes have a pleasant, hollow sound and are quieter than ceramic wind chimes. There are several companies that manufacture them. They do tend to be more expensive than standard wind chimes, but the sound quality is worth the extra money.

Do not use rhythm instruments that are obviously designed for children. Several toy companies manufacture unbreakable rhythm band sets, but they are of inferior quality in terms of sound and vibrotactile stimulation. They also look like children's instruments, and you want to be sure that the instruments you purchase are age-appropriate.

If you can afford it, you may consider purchasing a set of tone bells. Tone bells are similar to a xylophone except that the bells aren't attached to one another. If you have a set of tone bells, set out the black notes on a table and encourage the participant(s) to play them. The black notes make what is known as a "pentatonic scale." When playing pentatonic music, the song can begin or finish on any note in the scale and still sound complete, plus the notes all sound good when played together. It's a great way to encourage improvisation. You can play with the person or can allow the person to play the bells alone. If a second participant comes by who wants to play, s/he can; the music will still sound pleasant.

Mr. S. stood at the table playing the tone bells, which were arranged to create a pentatonic scale. He played intently for about five minutes. When the staff member came to stand next to him, he smiled and said, "This is nice!"

♪

Sing-Alongs

Persons who pace may not be able to sing all of the words to a song or may make up their own words. Like the Sensory Group, Walking Club participants may simply hum or listen to sing-alongs—that is still considered participation.

If you plan to use an instrument for accompaniment, it's best to play an instrument you can carry with you like a guitar, autoharp, or Omnichord. This way, you can mingle with the participants as they walk and you can observe the entire group.

Try to match the energy level of the group when you begin the sing-along. If the group is moving about quickly, play a fast song. If the group is quiet and moving slowly, play a quiet song. Meet the participants where they are; if you play a song that is too removed from their mood, you will have difficulty getting the group's attention.

Additional Ideas

Music boxes: Purchase some small, inexpensive music boxes. The participants can listen to them while walking.

Making instruments: Try making some musical instruments as a craft project. People who pace cannot sit down long enough to finish the project in one sitting, but may be able to finish the project over several days.

1. **Jingle bracelets:** Sew jingle bells onto a piece of cloth; sew Velcro to the ends.
2. **Jingle necklaces:** Thread jingle bells onto a piece of twine or plastic cord.
3. **Shakers:** Fill a small container (such as an empty, decorated toilet paper roll) with a handful of lentils and tape the container shut.
4. **Sand blocks:** Use a staplegun to attach medium-grain sandpaper to a pair of wood blocks approximately 5" x 3" x 1". Glue a wooden drawer pull on the opposite side.

One Final Note

If you're already using music with persons with dementia, I hope this book gave you a few new ideas. If you haven't used music with persons with dementia, I hope this book has encouraged you to try.

The bibliography and the resource list that follow contain much more information on music therapy, dementia, and activities. Good luck to you in your musical endeavors. I'll leave you with the words of an AFCC participant:

"No matter how lousy I feel, no matter how cranky I am, I always feel better after I sing. It releases something in you...I feel like whatever is bothering me, I let it all out."

♪

I know how she feels—it does the same thing for me. That's the beauty of music: its power is felt by both the listener and the performer. It's my hope that the power of music touches you as well as the person(s) with dementia with whom you work or live.

APPENDIX

Bibliography

Brotons, M. 1989. Paper presented at the "Gerontology in a New Age" seminar. 40th Annual Conference; National Association for Music Therapy, Inc., Kansas City, MO.

Butler, R. 1963. The life review: An interpretation of reminiscence in the aged. *Psychiatry* 26.1: 65-76.

Butler, R., and Lewis, M. 1982. *Aging and mental health: Positive psychosocial and biomedical approaches*. United States: C.V. Mosby and Co.

Clair, A., and Bernstein, B. 1990. A comparison of singing, vibrotactile stimulation and nonvibrotactile instrument playing responses in severely regressed patients of the Alzheimer's type. *Journal of Music Therapy* 27: 119-136.

Gibbons, A. 1977. Popular music preferences of older people. *Journal of Music Therapy* 14: 180-189.

Greenwald, M., and Salzberg, R. 1979. Vocal range assessment of geriatric clients. *Journal of Music Therapy* 16: 172-179.

Millard, K., and Smith, J. 1989. The influence of group singing therapy on the behavior of Alzheimer's disease patients. *Journal of Music Therapy* 26: 58-70.

Moreno, J. 1988. Multicultural music therapy: The world music connection. *Journal of Music Therapy* 25: 17-27.

Smith, D. 1988. The effect of enhanced higher frequencies on the musical preferences of older adults. *Journal of Music Therapy* 25: 62-72.

_______. 1989. Preference for differentiated frequency loudness levels in older adults' music listening. *Journal of Music Therapy* 26: 18-29.

Wylie, M. 1990. A comparison of the effects of old familiar songs, antique objects, historical summaries and general questions on the reminiscence of nursing home residents. *Journal of Music Therapy* 27: 2-12.

Music Therapy and Music in Geriatric Care

Barlett, J.C., and Snelus, P. 1980. Lifespan

memory for popular songs. *American Journal of Psychology* 93: 551-560.

Batcheller, J., and Monsour, S. 1972. *Music in recreation and leisure*. Dubuque, IA: Wm. C. Brown.

Bonny. H., and Savary, L. 1973. *Music and your mind*. New York: Harper and Row.

Bright, R. 1972. *Music in geriatric care*. New York: Musicgraphs.

______. 1981. *Practical planning in music therapy for the aged*. New York: Musicgraphs.

______. 1988. *Music therapy and the dementias*. Missouri: MMB Music, Inc.

Douglas, D. 1981. *Accent on rhythm: Music activities for the aged*. St. Louis, MO: MMB Music, Inc.

Gaston, E. Thayer, editor. 1968. *Music in therapy*. New York: MacMillan Publishing Co.

Gibbons, A.C. 1990. A review of literature for music development/education and music therapy with the elderly. *Music Therapy Perspectives* 5: 33-40.

Karras, B. 1985. *Down memory lane*. Mt. Airy, MD: ElderSong Publications, Inc.

______. 1990. *Mindstretchers*. Mt. Airy, MD: ElderSong Publications, Inc.

Katsch, S., and Merle-Fishman, C. 1985. *The music within you*. New York: Simon & Schuster.

Palmer, M.D. 1977. Music therapy in a comprehensive program of treatment and rehabilitation for the geriatric resident. *Journal of Music Therapy* 14: 190-197.

Riegler, J. 1980. Comparison of a reality orientation program for geriatric patients with and without music. *Journal of Music Therapy* 17: 26-33.

______. 1980. Most comfortable loudness level of geriatric patients as a function of Seashore loudness discrimination scores, detection threshold, age, sex, setting, and musical background. *Journal of Music Therapy* 17: 214-222.

Schweinsberg, M. 1981. Rhythm bands in the nursing home. *Activities, Adaptation and Aging* 1: 37-41.

Schulberg, C. 1981. *The music therapy sourcebook*. New York: Human Sciences Press.

Weissman, J.A. 1983. Planning music activities to meet needs and treatment goals of aged individuals in long-term care facilities. *Music Therapy* 3: 63-70.

Whitcomb, J.B., MA, CMT. 1989. Thanks for the memory. *American Journal of Alzheimer's Care and Related Disorders and Research* July/August: 22-33.

Readings in Dementia Care

Butler, R. 1984. How Alzheimer's became a public issue. *Generations* Fall, 1984, 33-35.

Caulking, M. 1988. *Design for dementia*. Maryland: National Health Publishing.

Cleland, M. 1988. *Prevention and management of aggressive behavior in the elderly*. Chicago: Good Samaritan Hospital.

Cohen, D., PhD., and Einsdorfer, C., M.D. 1986. *Loss of self*. New York: W.W. Norton & Co.

______. 1982. *Family handbook on Alzheimer's disease*. New York: Health Advancement Service.

Davis, R. 1989. *My journey Into Alzheimer's disease*. Wheaton, IL: Tyndale Publishers.

Feil, Naomi. 1984. Communicating with the confused elderly patient. *Geriatrics* 39, 176-189.

Fish, Sharon. 1990. *Alzheimer's: Caring for your loved one, caring for yourself.* Batavia, IL: Lion Publishing Corp.

Gwyther, L., ACSW. 1985. *Care of Alzheimer's patients: A manual for nursing home staff.* American Health Care Association and the Alzheimer's Association.

Mace, N., and Rabins, P. 1981. *The 36-hour day: A family guide to caring for persons with Alzheimer's disease, related dementing illnesses, and memory loss in later life*. Baltimore, MD: The Johns Hopkins University Press.

Nissenboim, S., & Vroman, C. 1988. *Interactions by design*. Missouri: Geri-Active Consultants.

Sincox, R., and Cohen, P. 1987. *Adapting the day care environment for the demented older adult*. Springfield, IL: Illinois Department on Aging.

Zgola, Jitka. 1987. *Doing things: A guide to programming activities for persons with Alzheimer's disease and related disorders*. Baltimore, MD: Johns Hopkins University Press.

Music Resources

Songbooks and Sing-Alongs

Javna, John. *The TV theme song sing-along book.* 1984. New York: St. Martin's Press.

Reader's Digest Songbooks. Reader's Digest Association, Inc. Pleasantville, NY 10570, (800) 431-1246. They also have record album collections of popular music. Here are the names of the books:

Popular Songs That Will Live Forever
Family Songbook of Faith and Joy
Merry Christmas Songbook
Unforgettable Musical Memories
Country and Western Songbook
Festival of Popular Songs
Remembering Yesterday's Hits
Family Songbook
Children's Songbook
Treasury of Best Loved Songs
The Easy Way to Play 100 Unforgettable Hits
Remembering the '50s

Stillman, Norton. 1971. *Trust me with your heart again: A fireside treasury of turn-of-the-century sheet music collected by Norton Stillman.* New York: Simon & Schuster. (212) 698-7000.

Tapes and Recordings

Bi-Folkal Productions, 809 Williamson Street, Madison, WI 53703, (608) 251-2818. Music and sing-along tapes and large print songbooks accompany each of the Bi-Folkal kits. Tapes and books may be purchased separately through their catalog, or check your local or regional library.

Recordings for Recovery, Michael Hoy, Executive Director, 413 Cherry, Midland, MI 48640, (517) 832-0784. R4R is a service of taped musical programs available to persons who are institutionalized, homebound, or otherwise limited by handicapping conditions. For a small yearly fee, subscribers are sent a listing of available tapes and are allowed to borrow as many as they would like to. The service is handled through the mail, much like the Talking Books program.

Radio Memories, P.O. Box 193, Yorktown Heights, NY 10598, (914) 245-6609. This company specializes in tapes of old radio shows.

Metro Golden Memories, 5425 W. Addison, Chicago, IL 60641, (312) 736-4133. Nostalgic recordings, tapes, photos, books, etc. Catalogs are available.

Musical Instruments

General Music Store, 19880 State Line Road, South Bend, IN 46637, (800) 348-5003.

Suzuki Musical Instruments, P.O. Box 261030, San Diego, CA 92126, (619) 566-9710.

Rhythm Band, Inc., P.O. Box 126, Ft. Worth, TX 76101, (817) 335-2561.

General Activity Resources

Hammatt Senior Products, P.O. Box 727, Mt. Vernon, WA 98273, (206) 428-5850.

Pickett Industries, P.O. Box 11000, Prescott, AZ 86304, (602) 778-1896.

Potentials Development, Inc., 775 Main St., Suite 604, Buffalo, NY 14203, (716) 842-2658.

Other Resources

American Association for Music Therapy, Inc., 66 Morris Avenue, Springfield, NJ 07081.

National Association for Music Therapy, Inc., 8455 Colesville Road, Suite 930, Silver Spring, MD 20910, (301) 589-3300. *The Journal of Music Therapy* and *Music Therapy Perspectives* are available through the NAMT at the subscription price of $24.00/yr.

Eldersong - A Newsletter for Those Using Music with Seniors, Beckie Karras, Publisher. ElderSong Publications, Inc., Box 74, Mt. Airy, MD 21771, (301) 829-0533.

Other resources available from ElderSong Publications, Inc.

Barbers, Cars, and Cigars: Activity Programming for Older Men

"Christmas With ElderSong"

Down Memory Lane

"Eldersong: The Music and Gerontology Newsletter"

Funny Bones Don't Get Arthritis: Humor for the Young at Heart

Hidden Treasures: Music and Memory Activities for People With Alzheimer's

Holiday Mind Joggers

Hooray for Hollywood: Trivia and Puzzles for Those Today Who Remember Yesterday

I Hear Memories!

Mind Joggers, Volumes 1 and 2

Mind Stretchers

Moments To Remember

Musings, Memories, and Make Believe

Puzzlers, Volumes 1 and 2

Say It With Music: Music Games and Trivia

"Sing-Along With ElderSong," Volumes 1 and 2

Trivia Treasury: Trivia and Word Games for Older Adults

What Do You Know? Trivia Fun and Activities for Seniors

Yesterdays: A Collection of Short Stories, Nostalgic Photographs, and Related Programming Materials for Seniors

ElderSong Publications, Inc. • P.O. Box 74, Mt. Airy, MD 21771 • 1-800-397-0533